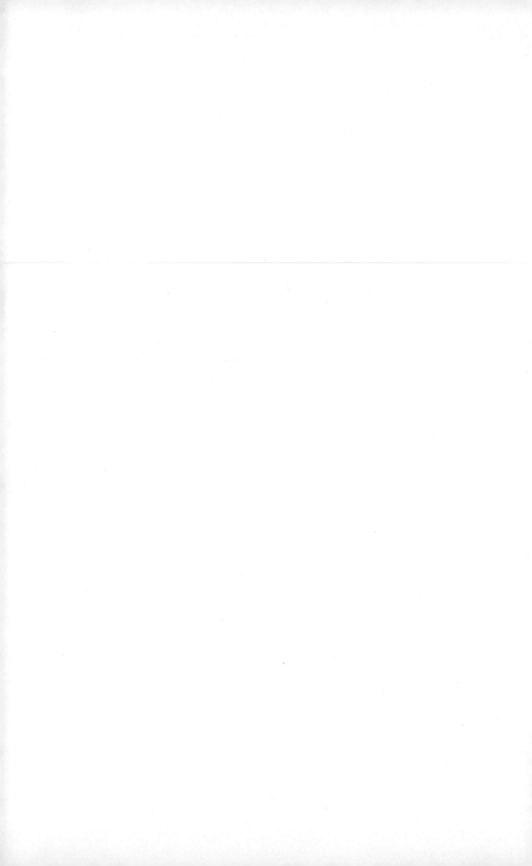

Mechanical Ventilation & Ventricular Assist Devices

Editors

JOHN J. MARINI
SRINIVAS MURALI

CRITICAL CARE CLINICS

www.criticalcare.theclinics.com

Consulting Editor
JOHN A. KELLUM

July 2018 • Volume 34 • Number 3

ELSEVIER

1600 John F. Kennedy Boulevard • Suite 1800 • Philadelphia, Pennsylvania, 19103-2899

http://www.theclinics.com

CRITICAL CARE CLINICS Volume 34, Number 3
July 2018 ISSN 0749-0704, ISBN-13: 978-0-323-61060-5

Editor: Colleen Dietzler
Developmental Editor: Casey Potter

Critical Care Clinics (ISSN: 0749-0704) is published quarterly by Elsevier Inc., 360 Park Avenue South, New York, NY 10010-1710. Months of issue are January, April, July, and October. Business and Editorial Offices: 1600 John F. Kennedy Blvd., Suite 1800, Philadelphia, PA 19103-2899. Customer Service Office: 6277 Sea Harbor Drive, Orlando, FL 32887-4800. Periodicals postage paid at New York, NY and additional mailing offices. Subscription prices are $234.00 per year for US individuals, $619.00 per year for US institution, $100.00 per year for US students and residents, $279.00 per year for Canadian individuals, $776.00 per year for Canadian institutions, $309.00 per year for international individuals, $776.00 per year for international institutions and $150.00 per year for Canadian and foreign students/residents. To receive student/resident rate, orders must be accompanied by name of affiliated institution, date of term, and the signature of program/residency coordinator on institution letterhead. Orders will be billed at individual rate until proof of status is received. Foreign air speed delivery is included in all *Clinics* subscription prices. All prices are subject to change without notice. POSTMASTER: Send address changes to *Critical Care Clinics*, Elsevier Periodicals Customer Service, 11830 Westline Industrial Drive, St. Louis, MO 63146. **Customer Service: 1-800-654-2452 (US). From outside of the US, call 1-314-447-8871. Fax: 1-314-447-8029. E-mail: journalscustomerservice-usa@ elsevier.com (for print support) or journalsonlinesupport-usa@elsevier.com (for online support).**

Reprints. For copies of 100 or more of articles in this publication, please contact the Commercial Reprints Department, Elsevier Inc., 360 Park Avenue South, New York, NY 10010-1710. Tel.: 212-633-3874; Fax: 212-633-3820; E-mail: reprints@elsevier.com.

Critical Care Clinics is also published in Spanish by Editorial Inter-Medica, Junin 917, 1er A, 1113, Buenos Aires, Argentina.

Critical Care Clinics is covered in *MEDLINE/PubMed (Index Medicus), EMBASE/Excerpta Medica, Current Concepts/ Clinical Medicine, ISI/BIOMED,* and *Chemical Abstracts.*

Printed in the United States of America.

Contributors

CONSULTING EDITOR

JOHN A. KELLUM, MD, MCCM
Professor of Critical Care Medicine, Medicine, Bioengineering and Clinical & Translational Science, Director, Center for Critical Care Nephrology, Vice Chair for Research, Department of Critical Care Medicine, University of Pittsburgh School of Medicine, Pittsburgh, Pennsylvania, USA

EDITORS

JOHN J. MARINI, MD
Professor of Medicine, Division of Pulmonary and Critical Care Medicine, University of Minnesota, Regions Hospital, St Paul, Minnesota, USA

SRINIVAS MURALI, MD
Professor of Medicine, Drexel University College of Medicine, System Director, Division of Cardiovascular Medicine, Department of Cardiothoracic Surgery, Co-Chair, Cardiovascular Institute, Allegheny Health Network, Pittsburgh, Pennsylvania, USA

AUTHORS

MASSIMO ANTONELLI, MD
Department of Anesthesia and Intensive Care, Fondazione Policlinico Universitario Agostino Gemelli, Università Cattolica del Sacro Cuore, Rome, Italy

STEPHEN BAILEY, MD
Department of Cardiothoracic Surgery, Cardiovascular Institute, Allegheny Health Network, Pittsburgh, Pennsylvania, USA

GIUSEPPE BELLO, MD
Department of Anesthesia and Intensive Care, Fondazione Policlinico Universitario Agostino Gemelli, Università Cattolica del Sacro Cuore, Rome, Italy

MICHELE BERTONI, MD
Department of Anesthesia, Critical Care and Emergency, Spedali Civili University Hospital, Brescia, Italy

RICHARD D. BRANSON, MSc, RRT, FCCM, FAARC
Professor of Surgery, Division of Trauma and Critical Care, University of Cincinnati, Cincinnati, Ohio, USA

LAURENT J. BROCHARD, MD
Program Director, Interdepartmental Division of Critical Care Medicine, University of Toronto, Keenan Research Centre for Biomedical Science, Li Ka Shing Knowledge Institute, St. Michael's Hospital, Toronto, Ontario, Canada

MITHUN CHAKRAVARTHY, MD
Coronary Artery Disease Program, Cardiovascular Institute, Allegheny General Hospital, Pittsburgh, Pennsylvania, USA

FRANCESCO CIPULLI, MD
Department of Anesthesiology, Emergency and Intensive Care Medicine, University of Göttingen, Göttingen, Germany; Dipartimento di Medicina e Chirurgia, Università degli Studi di Milano Bicocca, Milano, Italy

ELEONORA DUSCIO, MD
Department of Anesthesiology, Emergency and Intensive Care Medicine, University of Göttingen, Göttingen, Germany; Department of Pathophysiology and Transplantation, University of Milan, Milano, Italy

SITARAMESH EMANI, MD
Advanced Heart Failure and Cardiac Transplant, Division of Cardiovascular Medicine, The Ohio State University Wexner Medical Center, Columbus, Ohio, USA

LUCIANO GATTINONI, MD
Department of Anesthesiology and Intensive Care Medicine, University Hospital, Georg-August University of Göttingen, Department of Anesthesiology, Emergency and Intensive Care Medicine, University of Göttingen, Göttingen, Germany

VALENTINA GIAMMATTEO, MD
Department of Anesthesia and Intensive Care, Fondazione Policlinico Universitario Agostino Gemelli, Università Cattolica del Sacro Cuore, Rome, Italy

EWAN C. GOLIGHER, MD, PhD
Interdepartmental Division of Critical Care Medicine, University of Toronto, Division of Respirology, Department of Medicine, University Health Network, Toronto General Hospital, Toronto, Ontario, Canada

ALESSANDRA IONESCU MADDALENA, MD
Department of Anesthesia and Intensive Care, Fondazione Policlinico Universitario Agostino Gemelli, Università Cattolica del Sacro Cuore, Rome, Italy

MANREET K. KANWAR, MD
Section of Heart Failure/Transplant/MCS and Pulmonary Hypertension, Cardiovascular Institute, Allegheny Health Network, Associate Professor of Medicine, Temple University Lewis Katz School of Medicine, Pittsburgh, Pennsylvania, USA

PAUL H. MAYO, MD
Division of Pulmonary, Critical Care and Sleep Medicine, Donald and Barbara Zucker School of Medicine at Hofstra/Northwell, New Hyde Park, New York, USA

ONNEN MOERER, MD
Department of Anesthesiology and Intensive Care Medicine, University Hospital, Georg-August University of Göttingen, Göttingen, Germany

SRINIVAS MURALI, MD
Professor of Medicine, Drexel University College of Medicine, System Director, Division of Cardiovascular Medicine, Department of Cardiothoracic Surgery, Co-Chair, Cardiovascular Institute, Allegheny Health Network, Pittsburgh, Pennsylvania, USA

MARIA PATARROYO-APONTE, MD
Cardiovascular Institute, Allegheny General Hospital, Pittsburgh, Pennsylvania, USA

TÀI PHAM, MD, PhD
Interdepartmental Division of Critical Care Medicine, University of Toronto, Keenan
Research Centre for Biomedical Science, Li Ka Shing Knowledge Institute, St. Michael's
Hospital, Toronto, Ontario, Canada

THOMAS PIRAINO, RRT
Department of Respiratory Therapy, St. Michael's Hospital, Toronto, Ontario, Canada

MICHAEL QUINTEL, MD
Department of Anesthesiology and Intensive Care Medicine, University Hospital,
Georg-August University of Göttingen, Department of Anesthesiology, Emergency
and Intensive Care Medicine, University of Göttingen, Göttingen, Germany

AMRESH RAINA, MD, FACC
Associate Director, Pulmonary Hypertension Program, Section of Heart
Failure/Transplant/MCS and Pulmonary Hypertension, Cardiovascular Institute,
Allegheny General Hospital, Assistant Professor of Medicine, Temple University
School of Medicine, Pittsburgh, Pennsylvania, USA

FEDERICA ROMITTI, MD
Department of Anesthesiology and Intensive Care Medicine, University Hospital,
Georg-August University of Göttingen, Department of Anesthesiology, Emergency
and Intensive Care Medicine, University of Göttingen, Göttingen, Germany

ANNIA SCHREIBER, MD
Respiratory Intensive Care Unit and Pulmonary Rehabilitation Unit, Istituti Clinici
Scientifici Maugeri, Scientific Institute of Pavia, Pavia, Italy

KEYUR B. SHAH, MD
Associate Professor of Medicine, Division of Cardiology, Department of Internal Medicine,
Advanced Heart Failure and Transplantation, Pauley Heart Center, Virginia
Commonwealth University, Richmond, Virginia, USA

MELISSA C. SMALLFIELD, MD
Assistant Professor of Medicine, Division of Cardiology, Department of Internal Medicine,
Advanced Heart Failure and Transplantation, Pauley Heart Center, Virginia
Commonwealth University, Richmond, Virginia, USA

INNA TCHOUKINA, MD
Assistant Professor of Medicine, Division of Cardiology, Department of Internal Medicine,
Advanced Heart Failure and Transplantation, Pauley Heart Center, Virginia
Commonwealth University, Richmond, Virginia, USA

IRENE TELIAS, MD
Interdepartmental Division of Critical Care Medicine, University of Toronto, Keenan
Research Centre for Biomedical Science, Li Ka Shing Knowledge Institute, St. Michael's
Hospital, Toronto, Ontario, Canada

MASAKI TSUKASHITA, MD
Department of Cardiothoracic Surgery, Cardiovascular Institute, Allegheny General
Hospital, Pittsburgh, Pennsylvania, USA

ETIENO U. UMOBONG, MD
Division of Pulmonary, Critical Care and Sleep Medicine, Donald and Barbara Zucker
School of Medicine at Hofstra/Northwell, New Hyde Park, New York, USA

FRANCESCO VASQUES, MD
Department of Anesthesiology, Emergency and Intensive Care Medicine, University of Göttingen, Göttingen, Germany; Department of Medicine (DMED), Anesthesia and Intensive Care Unit, Padua University Hospital, Padua, Italy

TAKESHI YOSHIDA, MD, PhD
Interdepartmental Division of Critical Care Medicine, University of Toronto, Keenan Research Centre for Biomedical Science, Li Ka Shing Knowledge Institute, St. Michael's Hospital, Translational Medicine, Departments of Critical Care Medicine and Anesthesia, Hospital for Sick Children, University of Toronto, Toronto, Ontario, Canada

Contents

Section I: Mechanical Ventilation

prolongs ventilator dependence, predisposing patients to nosocomial complications and death. Limb muscle weakness persists for months after discharge from intensive care and results in poor long-term functional status and quality of life. Major mechanisms of muscle injury include critical illness polymyoneuropathy, sepsis, pharmacologic exposures, metabolic derangements, and excessive muscle loading and unloading. The diaphragm may become weak because of excessive unloading (leading to atrophy) or because of excessive loading (either concentric or eccentric) owing to insufficient ventilator assistance.

Closed loop control of mechanical ventilation is routine and operates behind the ventilator interface. Reducing caregiver interactions is neither an advantage for the patient or the staff. Automated systems causing lack of situational awareness of the intensive care unit are a concern. Along with autonomous systems must come monitoring and displays of patients' current condition and response to therapy. Alert notifications for sudden escalation of therapy are required to ensure patient safety. Automated ventilation is useful in remote settings in the absence of experts. Whether automated ventilation will be accepted in large academic medical centers remains to be seen.

Noninvasive ventilation (NIV) has assumed a central role in the treatment of select patients with acute respiratory failure owing to exacerbated chronic obstructive pulmonary disease or acute cardiogenic pulmonary edema. Recent advances in the understanding of physiologic aspects of NIV application through different interfaces and ventilator settings have led to improved patient-machine interaction, enhancing favorable NIV outcome. In recent years, the growing role of NIV in the acute care setting has led to the development of technical innovations to overcome the problems related to gas leakage and dead space, improving the quality of the devices and optimizing ventilation modes.

Extracorporeal gas exchange is increasingly used for various indications. Among these are refractory acute respiratory failure, including the acute respiratory distress syndrome, and the avoidance of ventilator-induced lung injury by enabling lung-protective ventilation. In addition, extracorporeal gas exchange allows the treatment of hypercapnic respiratory failure while helping to unload the respiratory muscles and avoid intubation and invasive ventilation, as well as facilitating weaning from the ventilator. These indications are based on a reasonable physiologic rationale but must be weighed against the costs and complications associated with the technique. This article summarizes current evidence and indications for extracorporeal gas exchange.

Section II: Ventricular Assist Devices

A Targeted Management Approach to Cardiogenic Shock   423

Mithun Chakravarthy, Masaki Tsukashita, and Srinivas Murali

> Cardiogenic shock is a clinical syndrome characterized by low cardiac output
> and sustained tissue hypoperfusion resulting in end-organ dysfunction and
> death. In-hospital mortality rates range from 50% to 60%. Urgent diagnosis
> and timely transfer to a tertiary or quaternary medical facility with critical care
> management capabilities and multidisciplinary shock teams is a must to in-
> crease survival. Aggressive, hemodynamically guided medical management
> with careful monitoring of clinical and hemodynamic parameters with timely
> use of appropriate mechanical circulatory support devices is often neces-
> sary. As treatment options evolve, prospective randomized controlled trials
> are needed to define best practices that define superior clinical outcomes.

Prevention and Treatment of Right Ventricular Failure During Left Ventricular
Assist Device Therapy   439

Amresh Raina and Maria Patarroyo-Aponte

> Left ventricular assist devices (LVADs) are increasingly used for the treat-
> ment of end-stage heart failure. Right ventricular (RV) failure after LVAD im-
> plantation is an increasingly common clinical problem, occurring in
> patients early after continuous flow LVAD implant. RV failure is associated
> with a substantial increase in post-LVAD morbidity and mortality. RV failure
> can be predicted using preoperative hemodynamic, clinical, and echocar-
> diographic variables and a variety of risk prediction algorithms. However,
> RV failure may also develop owing to unanticipated intraoperative or peri-
> operative factors. Early recognition and treatment are critical in terms of
> mitigating the impact of RV failure on post-LVAD outcomes.

Device Management and Flow Optimization on Left Ventricular Assist
Device Support   453

Inna Tchoukina, Melissa C. Smallfield, and Keyur B. Shah

> The authors discuss principles of continuous flow left ventricular assist de-
> vice (LVAD) operation, basic differences between the axial and centrifugal
> flow designs and hemodynamic performance, normal LVAD physiology,
> and device interaction with the heart. Systematic interpretation of LVAD
> parameters and recognition of abnormal patterns of flow and pulsatility
> on the device interrogation are necessary for clinical assessment of the pa-
> tient. Optimization of pump flow using LVAD parameters and echocardio-
> graphic and hemodynamics guidance are reviewed.

Complications of Durable Left Ventricular Assist Device Therapy   465

Sitaramesh Emani

> Patients with heart failure on durable left ventricular assist device support
> experience improved survival, quality of life, and exercise capacity. The

complication rate, however, remains unacceptably high, although it has declined with improvements in pump design, better patient selection, and greater understanding of the pump physiology and flow dynamics. Most complications are categorized as those related to the pump-patient interface or those related to patient physiology. It is hoped that further engineering progress, and better patient selection through risk stratification, will allow for left ventricular assist device to be totally biocompatible and perform effectively, without affecting biology and homeostasis of the different organ systems.

Manreet K. Kanwar, Stephen Bailey, and Srinivas Murali

The clinical use of left ventricular assist devices (LVADs) in the growing epidemic of heart failure has improved quality of life and long-term survival for this otherwise devastating disease. The current generation of commercially available devices offers a smaller profile that simplifies surgical implantation, a design that optimizes blood flow characteristics, with less adverse events and improved durability than their predecessors. Despite this, the risk for adverse events remains significant, as do burdens for patients and their caregivers. Appropriate patient selection remains key to optimal LVAD outcomes.

CRITICAL CARE CLINICS

THE CLINICS ARE AVAILABLE ONLINE!
Access your subscription at:
www.theclinics.com

Section I: Mechanical Ventilation

Preface

Mechanical Ventilation

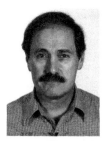

John J. Marini, MD
Editor

Mechanical ventilation, the ability to artificially compensate for life-threatening failure of respiratory function, is often considered the signature technology of intensive care medicine. Unchanging needs for providing effective life support with minimized risk and optimized comfort will continue to be the principal objectives of applying this powerful and steadily improving technology. Important lessons acquired over many years of intensive care unit practice have brought us closer to meeting those goals, even as advances in instrumentation facilitate putting this hard-won knowledge into action. Rising demand in the face of economic constraints is likely to drive future innovations focused on reducing the need for user input, automating multielement protocols, and carefully monitoring the patient for progress and complications at an early stage. With passing time, the goals of ventilatory support have been extended and refined to include not only effective gas exchange and offloading of the ventilatory burden but also minimized iatrogenesis, avoidance of lingering disability, and improved coordination between the patient's innate neural controller and the response of machine-delivered breathing cycles. Dramatic improvements in extracorporeal gas exchange now complement those occurring with traditional ventilation. The capacity of mechanical ventilators to ventilate and oxygenate effectively has steadily improved, while the caregiver has become aware of its potential to promote infection, hemodynamic consequences, ventilator-induced lung injury, and diaphragmatic dysfunction that may contribute to, or perhaps even initiate, post–intensive care syndrome. Once an inherently uncomfortable process that invariably required deep sedation, airway intubation, and even paralysis to maintain, "artificial ventilation" provided by modern machines and extracorporeal devices now offers diverse options (noninvasive as well as invasive) to reduce breathing work load, reduce discomfort, improve oxygen exchange, enhance coordination, and avoid ventilator-induced lung injury.

As an editor of this issue on advances in respiratory support, I have been privileged to invite exceptional contributors to recount the important lessons we have learned

Crit Care Clin 34 (2018) xiii–xiv
https://doi.org/10.1016/j.ccc.2018.04.001
0749-0704/18/© 2018 Published by Elsevier Inc.

during the positive pressure ventilation era, describe current developments, and suggest remaining problems and innovative approaches that point toward future progress. Due to unforeseen circumstances, the contribution of Marcelo Amato to this issue on mechanical ventilation will be published in an upcoming issue of *Critical Care Clinics*. The range of selected topics reflects the most current, clinically relevant issues as well as the innovative thinking likely to meet those clinical challenges going forward. I am sincerely indebted to each of these outstanding leaders and educators of our field for accepting my invitation.

John J. Marini, MD
Division of Pulmonary and
Critical Care Medicine
University of Minnesota
Regions Hospital
MS 11203B
640 Jackson Street
St Paul, MN 55101, USA

E-mail address:
marin002@umn.edu

Critical Care Airway Management

Etieno U. Umobong, MD*, Paul H. Mayo, MD

KEYWORDS

- Endotracheal intubation • Complications • Quality improvement • Difficult airway
- MACOCHA score

KEY POINTS

- Urgent endotracheal intubation is associated with a variety of dangerous complications.
- Rapid sequence intubation and graded sequence intubation are both effective means of induction during endotracheal intubation.
- Both direct laryngoscopy and video laryngoscopy are effective means to guide endotracheal intubation.
- Preoxygenation is an important element to reduce risk of severe desaturation during urgent endotracheal intubation.
- Focused training in critical care airway management may reduce the complication rate.

INTRODUCTION

Urgent endotracheal intubation (UEI) in the critically ill patient is performed outside the operating theater by emergency medicine personnel and by intensivists with a variety of training backgrounds that include medicine, surgery, and anesthesiology. This article reviews some issues related to critical care airway management. These include complications of UEI, identification of the difficult airway, rapid sequence intubation (RSI) versus graded sedation intubation (GSI), direct laryngoscopy (DL) versus video laryngoscopy (VL), utility and techniques of preoxygenation, utility of gastric ultrasonography, and improvement in safety of UEI.

UEI is a high-risk procedure with a variety of complications: oxygen desaturation, hypotension, cardiac arrest, and death may occur related to UEI as well as difficulty with endotracheal tube insertion, airway/injury, and esophageal intubation. Although some investigators focus on measurements of the outcome of UEI that emphasize

---

Disclosure Statement: The authors have no financial disclosures or conflicts of interest to declare.

Division of Pulmonary, Critical Care and Sleep Medicine, Zucker School of Medicine at Hofstra/Northwell, 410 Lakeville Road, Suite 107, New Hyde Park, NY 11040, USA
* Corresponding author.
E-mail address: eumobong@northwell.edu

the time and number of passes required to insert the endotracheal tube, more sophisticated methods of assessing the quality of UEI focus on physiologic endpoints during the procedure, such as blood pressure and oxygen saturation. Heterogeneous study populations undergo UEI, so it is difficult to compare results of interventions between studies. This difficulty is compounded by the heterogeneity of training background and experience of the clinicians who perform UEI. The multiplicity of intubation devices is a challenge when comparing endotracheal intubation outcomes. This article reviews some of the recent literature about UEI and represents the opinions of the authors, who are critical care specialists with extensive frontline experience in UEI.

COMPLICATIONS OF URGENT ENDOTRACHEAL INTUBATION

Although successful insertion of the endotracheal tube is the goal of UEI, a primary concern is maintenance of gas exchange and hemodynamic function throughout the procedure. Physiologic alterations characteristic of a patient with critical illness, side effects of pharmacologic agents, time pressure, and operator inexperience combine to increase the risk of severe desaturation and hypotension during UEI. Jaber and colleagues[1] reported a high rate of severe complications during UEI, with a focus on physiologically relevant measurements, reporting at least 1 severe complication occurring in 28% of patients. This group went on to define hypotension and acute respiratory failure as independent risk factors for complicated UEI, noting that supervision by an experienced physician helped mitigate this risk. The formal definition of these complications provides the field with a useful method to report and compare outcomes of UEI (**Box 1**). In a large prospective multicenter study De Jong and colleagues,[2] using these standard definitions of complications, reported a 35% rate of severe complications during UEI. This study likely represents an accurate real-world

---

Box 1
Standardized definitions for complications of urgent endotracheal intubation

Life-threatening complications of UEI

- Severe hypoxemia (<80% oxygen saturation)
- Severe hemodynamic collapse (systolic blood pressure <60 mm Hg or systolic blood pressure <90 mm Hg after 500 mL–1000 mL fluid bolus >30 minutes after intubation or requiring pressors)
- Cardiac arrest
- Death

Other immediate complications of UEI

- Difficult intubation ($\geq$3 intubation attempts or lasting >10 minutes)
- Cardiac arrhythmia
- Esophageal intubation
- Agitation
- Aspiration
- Dental injury

Data from Jaber S, Amraoui J, Lefrant JY, et al. Clinical practice and risk factors for immediate complications of endotracheal intubation in the intensive care unit: a prospective, multiple-center study. Crit Care Med 2006;34:2355–61.

---

number, because it was derived from a total of 34 centers having a wide range of capability. Single-center studies have reported much lower rates, but these may reflect local expertise in UEI.

Key to any program designed to improve the quality of UEI is ongoing assessment of complication rates. The work of Jaber and colleagues[1] allows a UEI team to measure complication rates using a standard set of parameters. The authors encourage wider use of these standardized physiologic definitions of complications for identification of local quality issues, for determination of the effect of quality-improvement projects designed to reduce complication rate, and for research purposes.

IDENTIFICATION OF THE DIFFICULT AIRWAY IN URGENT ENDOTRACHEAL INTUBATION

The term, *difficult airway*, is used to describe endotracheal intubation where anatomic considerations make visualization of the vocal cords and insertion of the endotracheal tube unusually challenging. The anesthesiology community has developed guidelines that are useful in identifying patients who will be difficult to intubate in the operating room. These have been adapted to UEI. De Jong and colleagues[2] defined a difficult airway in UEI as requiring more than 3 attempts at endotracheal tube insertion and/or more than 10 minutes for successful endotracheal intubation. With this definition, they reported an 11% incidence of difficult airways (N = 1000 UEI from 26 centers). These data were used to derive a scoring system (the Mallampati score, apnea, cervical spine mobility, mouth opening, coma, hypoxemia, and nonanesthesiology [MACOCHA] score) useful for identifying patients with a potential difficult airway (**Table 1**). The scoring system was subsequently validated on 400 patients from 18 additional medical centers.

If the MACOCHA score is low, the likelihood of a difficult airway is low; if it is high, a patient has augmented risk of a difficult airway, with a higher score indicating a higher probability of a difficult airway, leading to the recommendation that

> It is prudent to be prepared for a difficult intubation, even if the intubation is finally not difficult.[2]

There are practical problems with measurement of the MACOCHA score in all patients requiring UEI. A major contributor to the final score is the Mallampati score. Many critically ill patients are unable to perform the basic requirement for Mallampati

Table 1
Factors used to formulate the MACOCHA score

Factors	Points
Mallampati score III or IV	5
Obstructive sleep apnea	2
Reduced mobility of cervical spine	1
Limited mouth opening <3 cm	1
Coma	1
Severe hypoxemia <80%	1
Nonanesthesiology trained	1
Total	12

From De Jong A, Molinari N, Terzi N, et al. Early identification of patients at risk for difficult intubation in the intensive care unit: development and validation of the MACOCHA score in a multicenter cohort study. Am J Respir Crit Care Med 2013;187:832–9; with permission.

score, which is volitional opening of the mouth while in sitting position. The maneuver has some value when performed in the nonstandard supine position, but many patients cannot perform volitional mouth opening even when supine. Mouth opening and cervical spine flexibility may be difficult to ascertain in a critically ill patient, yet these are also elements of the scoring system required to predict the difficult airway.

The MACOCHA score only has utility if a patient is able to perform the maneuvers required to determine it. One means of improving its application is to attempt to routinely measure it in all patients who come under care of the critical care team, regardless of any immediate need for UEI. Inevitably, there are some patients in whom the full score cannot be obtained.

Although not reported in the MACOCHA study, it is likely that a majority of UEIs were performed with DL. It is possible that if VL is used as the primary device to accomplish endotracheal tube insertion, the rate and risk factors for difficult airway are redefined.

Mosier and colleagues[3] have reviewed the "physiologically difficult airway," a category in which risk of severe hypotension, hypoxemia, and death is increased during UEI, independent of anatomic constraints. Risk factors include the presence of pre-procedure hypotension, hypoxemia, severe metabolic acidosis, and right ventricular failure. Methods have been proposed to reduce complications in this vulnerable population (**Table 2**).

The a priori identification of the difficult airway is important for several reasons:

1. It allows the UEI team to prepare for a difficult intubation. This might include immediate availability at bedside of advanced airway devices (eg, video laryngoscope, rigid fiberoptic stylet, flexible fiberoptic bronchoscope, transtracheal jet ventilator catheter, tracheostomy equipment, and supraglottic airway).
2. It allows the UEI team to preposition personnel with expert-level capability at airway management at the bedside. The wide variability of complication rates for UEI suggests that operator experience may be a major factor in outcomes of UEI.[4]
3. The occurrence of a difficult airway during UEI is associated with a higher complication rate compared with a routine airway, because the rates of hypotension, desaturation, and death during UEI are higher with difficult intubation than with routine intubation.[2] Although several groups have reported that specific interventions have

Table 2
Summary of factors that predict physiologically difficult airway

Hypoxemia	• Preoxygenation • Consider inclusion of apneic oxygenation via nasal cannula to prolong safe apneic time until tube insertion.
Hypotension	• Early use of vasopressors prior to induction especially if systolic blood pressure <100 prior to induction • Norepinephrine is preferred.
Severe metabolic acidosis	• Consider graded sedation induction to maintain respiratory drive, especially in patient with high minute ventilation. • Trial of NIPPV while correcting underlying metabolic derangements and to estimate minute volume for ventilator setting
Right ventricular failure	• Bedside echocardiography to assess right ventricular function • When possible, RV afterload reduction agents like inhaled nitric oxide and epoprostenol should be used prior to intubation. • Preoxygenation and vasopressor support are essential.

Data from Mosier JM, Joshi R, Hypes C, et al. The physiologically difficult airway. West J Emerg Med 2015;16:1109–17.

resulted in reduction of complications of UEI, to date there is no definitive study that indicates whether specific interventions that target recognition of patients with difficult airways would result in a lower rate of complications in that specific population. Intuitively, this is likely to be the case.

RAPID SEQUENCE INTUBATION VERSUS GRADED SEDATION INTUBATION FOR URGENT ENDOTRACHEAL INTUBATION

Two pharmacologic strategies are used during UEI: RSI and GSI. With RSI, the team uses a sedative agent(s) to achieve unconsciousness in a patient followed by use of a neuromuscular blocking drug, most commonly the depolarizing agent succinylcholine, to achieve paralysis. This is followed by an attempt at endotracheal tube insertion. If there is a contraindication to succinylcholine, a short-acting nondepolarizing agent is an alternative. The advantages of RSI are that paralysis of a patient is presumed to result in optimal visualization of the vocal chords due to absence of patient movement and reduced difficulty of insertion of endotracheal tube through the cords given their lack of respirophasic movement or vocal cord spasm.

RSI is well suited to endotracheal intubation in the operating room; patients are fully assessed for difficult airway risk, intubating conditions are optimal, anesthesiologists are highly skilled at intubation, and patients usually have relatively normal respiratory physiology. Preoxygenation results in a large reservoir of oxygen in thoracic compartment, so that without agitation to consume it, time from apnea to patient desaturation is prolonged.

Standard anesthesiology practice allows identification of a patient who is likely to be difficult to intubate. Such patients are triaged to awake intubation technique using fiberoptic methods. If an anesthesiologist encounters unanticipated difficulty with endotracheal intubation while using RSI, the patient receives bag-valve-mask (BVM) ventilation/oxygenation until the induction agents wear off. This may not be feasible with non-RSI UEI. The rare complication of lethal hyperkalemia from succinylcholine may be avoided in scheduled surgical cases utilizing RSI because the patient can be screened for risk factors before use of the agent.

The downsides to RSI for UEI are summarized as follows:

1. The use of a paralytic agent implies that an operator has a high level of first-pass success, and, failing this, that the team is able to provide adequate BVM for ventilation/oxygenation while setting up for the second attempt. Although the safe use of RSI is predicated on a high level of success with first-pass at endotracheal tube insertion, it may not always be possible to identify a difficult airway during setup for UEI. Lacking the ability to accurately assess difficulty of endotracheal intubation using standard methods available to the elective operating room anesthesiologist, the risk of difficult intubation is increased in UEI. Even if the critical care team identifies a difficult airway during setup for UEI, a patient can be so unstable that fiberoptic intubation may not be feasible. If the critical care team fails on first-pass attempt, they are faced with an apneic patient who may have major gas exchange abnormality. There is no "wake up and back out" option with UEI with RSI.
2. If a team fails with the initial intubation attempt, the bailout is to provide BVM oxygenation while the team sets up for the second attempt. If a patient has severe underlying lung disease (pneumonia, acute respiratory distress syndrome, or airflow obstruction) or poor facial anatomy, this reoxygenation attempt may fail. Desaturation during apnea may be rapid in the face of lung disease that commonly is the indication for UEI. The situation then devolves into increasingly desperate attempts at intubation followed by further failed attempts at BVM use.

3. A rare complication of succinylcholine is lethal hyperkalemia. The UEI team may not be able to identify risk factors for this event in an emergent situation. Although use a nondepolarizing agent, such as rocuronium, removes this risk, the longer duration of action of this agent is a major disadvantage compared with the short duration of succinylcholine.

4. Because the success of RSI is predicated on first-pass success of endotracheal intubation, it requires that an operator be highly skilled. This skill level is typical for a fully trained anesthesiologist but may not be the case for the non–anesthesiology-trained intensivist or emergency medicine clinician. This lack of experience is a problem particular in the United States, where a majority of intensivists do not have from anesthesiology training backgrounds, unlike in Europe. Buis and colleagues[5] reported that the number of intubations required to achieve a 90% success rate within 2 passes is greater than 50 for elective operating room intubations whereas the risk of difficult intubation increased 20-fold in UEI. Bernhard and colleagues[6] studied the learning curve for UEI amongst anesthesiology residents. After 200 procedures, an average of 1.6 attempts were still required for successful endotracheal intubation whereas 83% of attempts were successful on first-pass. This indicates that even 200 completed UEIs may not result in the skill level required for high RSI safety. Although the anesthesiology trainee may achieve these numbers, typical critical care medicine or emergency medicine training programs in the United States do not provide their trainees with a sufficient number of UEIs to approach anesthesiology-level capability in endotracheal intubation. Inadequate skill level at endotracheal tube placement increases the risk of converting a UEI using RSI to a scenario of cannot bag/cannot intubate.

GSI does not include the use of a neuromuscular blocking agent. Instead, the team uses sedative agent(s) to establish adequate intubating conditions while allowing a patient to maintain spontaneous breathing. The patient can continue to maintain gas exchange throughout the process of insertion of the endotracheal tube. The patient receives high-flow oxygen supplementation designed to meet all inspiratory flow requirements, entraining an Fio_2 approaching 1.0 during the procedure. Oxygen may be delivered by high-flow nasal source; directed insufflation of oxygen into the mouth; or, with high-risk patients, applying nasal noninvasive positive pressure ventilation (NIPPV) with use of the video laryngoscope. One group has described use of nasal NIPPV with simultaneous fiberoptic endotracheal intubation technique.[7] GSI emphasizes maintenance of oxygen saturation throughout the procedure as a primary safety endpoint rather than the speed or rate of first-pass success for tube insertion. The downsides to GSI are summarized as follows:

1. The sedative agents used for GSI, such as propofol, benzodiazepines, or opiates, cause vasoplegia. This effect is exaggerated with sepsis and/or hypovolemia and by application of positive pressure ventilation. The best strategy to counteract the predictable vasoplegic effect of GSI agents is the early aggressive use of vasopressor agents, such as norepinephrine, to avoid hypotension. The preemptive use of vasopressors is appropriate in high-risk patients; before the sedative agent is given, the patient is placed on the vasopressor to block hypotension from occurring. The defense of blood pressure is a primary goal of GSI, as is the defense of oxygen saturation, with the endotracheal intubation being a secondary goal. Koenig and colleagues[8] reported the safe use of propofol as the sedating agent for UEI in 409 patients with a rate of hypotension similar to large studies of UEI that used predominately RSI technique.

2. The time required for UEI may be longer with GSI compared with RSI. Sequential doses of sedative agent titrated to achieve adequate sedation may take more time than the dosing regimen required for RSI. The time required to perform the actual endotracheal tube insertion may be somewhat longer with GSI than with RSI, because patients are breathing during the procedure. This prolongation is generally well tolerated. Using GSI, Koenig and colleagues[8] report a rate of desaturation during UEI that is comparable to that reported with RSI.

There is no randomized controlled trial comparing the 2 induction methods. Several large studies have documented the successful use of RSI for UEI, particularly in the emergency medicine setting. Results are usually reported in terms of success, speed, and number of attempts required for intubation without report of the important physiologic endpoints of blood pressure and oxygen saturation. Combined with the heterogeneity of the patient population and skill of the operator, it is difficult to compare the results of these studies with those of studies that focus on physiologic endpoints. Jaber and colleagues, a group with an anesthesiology background, have performed landmark studies that report on physiologic endpoints while favoring RSI. A series of reports from a group that uses GSI indicates that the rate of complications using the standards set by Jaber and colleagues[1] are similar to those reported by groups that use RSI.[8–10]

Lacking a definitive RCT comparing GSI to RSI, the authors speculate that the major factor in assuring safety of UEI lies not in the induction technique but on the use of an organized team approach to maintain a safe operational environment. The authors advise critical care teams that RSI requires a high level of skill at the physical actions required for endotracheal intubation and that quality assessment includes tracking physiologic endpoints and not just success of endotracheal tube placement. Clinical equipoise exists between GSI and RSI pending further research.

DIRECT LARYNGOSCOPY VERSUS VIDEO LARYNGOSCOPY FOR URGENT ENDOTRACHEAL INTUBATION

DL is a well-established method for endotracheal intubation, both in the operating room and for UEI. An attractive alternative is the VL. In considering whether 1 device has advantage over another in elective operating room airway management, Lewis and colleagues,[11] in a Cochrane meta-analysis, concluded that, although there was no overall outcome difference between the 2 devices, VL may have specific utility in cases where DL has failed and for difficult airway management.

Is there advantage of 1 device over the other for UEI? In a meta-analysis that focused on UEI, De Jong and colleagues[12] compared DL to VL. VL was associated with a reduced risk of difficult intubation, better glottic visualization, reduced esophageal intubation, and increased first-pass success. In counterpoint, Huang and colleagues[13] concluded from a meta-analysis that there exists no inherent difference between the 2 devices when used for UEI. The contradictory literature on VL may reflect heterogeneity of patient populations, varying skill levels of the operators, different designs of VL, different techniques for use of the VL, and experiences of the team with the 2 devices.

It is likely that an expert anesthesiologist will be successful with either instrument while favoring VL for the difficult airway. The situation may be different for an intensivist who lacks anesthesiology training and extensive experience with DL. VL has been compared with DL for UEI performed by nonanesthesiology intensivists, including pulmonary critical care fellows. Mosier and colleagues[14] reported use of VL by critical care fellows compared with DL improved glottis visualization, first-pass success rate, and decreased esophageal intubation rate among critical care fellows. Kory and colleagues[15] reported on both retrospective and prospective study design that VL was superior to DL for first-pass success and reduction of esophageal intubation.[16] Lakticova and colleagues,[9] with a before and after study design, reported that the use of VL by pulmonary critical care medicine fellows was associated with reduced rate of difficult intubation and esophageal intubation without increased risk of failure of physiologic endpoints. These results are contradicted by Lascarrou and colleagues,[17] who reported the rate of serious complications during UEI using VL was higher that with DL. This study has methodological problems that include use of a nonstandard stylet, a VL different in design from those used in other studies, and the use of bougies.

The learning curve for VL has not been determined by formal study. Repetitive deliberate practice on task trainers seems an effective means of preparing pulmonary critical care medicine fellows for actual UEI. This suggests that the learning curve for VL is considerably steeper than for DL. Ambrosio and colleagues[18] used difficult airway simulated manikins to demonstrate the learnability and ease of use of VL for novices. Their cohort of 40 first-year residents using the VL versus DL had a 100% intubation rate versus 47.4%, respectively, with intubation times 67s versus 23s. This is a major advantage for an intensivist trainee who is not able to achieve full competence in use of the DL during typical fellowship training in the United States, because full anesthesiology training is required to meet the number of procedures required for full competence in use of the DL for UEI.

PREOXYGENATION TECHNIQUES FOR URGENT ENDOTRACHEAL INTUBATION

Avoidance of hypoxemia is a primary objective during UEI. Severe hypoxemia is a common occurrence during UEI; De Jong and colleagues[2] reported a 35% rate of severe desaturation during UEI (>80 saturation). For an elective operating case, preoxygenation is readily achieved by denitrogenation of the functional residual capacity (FRC), thereby providing patients with a substantial oxygen reservoir, especially for apneic patients. Effective preoxygenation of a patient with normal lung function blocks desaturation during apnea for several minutes during the process of endotracheal elective operating room intubation.

Some patients who require UEI have normal lung function (eg, patients with neuro-injury and metabolic disarray). Preoxygenation is straightforward in this population using techniques that are used in the operating room. Patients with severe lung disease, such as acute respiratory distress syndrome, severe pneumonia, or infiltrative lung disease, are at high risk of desaturation during UEI. Even with effective denitrogenation, the shunt physiology that accompanies severe parenchymal lung disease of this type results in a short time to desaturation during apnea. The efficiency of preoxygenation in patients with hypoxemic respiratory failure is difficult to determine by O_2 saturation alone. This requires measurement of the Pao_2, which is impractical during a high-risk UEI. Even if the team is able to raise the O_2 saturation to 100%, the Pao_2 remains unknown.

Several methods have been studied to improve preoxygenation for UEI. Mort[19] reported that use of BVM with Fio_2 for 4 minutes or 8 minutes was marginally effective in preoxygenating patients requiring UEI.[20] Baillard and colleagues[21] reported that 3 minutes of NIPPV using a tight-fitting full-face mask with positive end-expiratory pressure (PEEP) of 5 cm H_2O was more effective than BVM preoxygenation. Sakles and colleagues[22] and Miguel-Montanes and colleagues[23] both reported that high-flow nasal O_2 (60 L/min) was effective in attenuating desaturation during UEI in patients with mild to moderate hypoxemia, although Vourc'h and colleagues[24] found this approach was not effective in patients with severe hypoxemia. High-flow nasal O_2 may improve saturation by replenishment of O_2 taken up from the lungs during apnea as well as by providing some degree of PEEP that reduces risk of derecruitment during apnea. Jaber and colleagues[25] described a protocol using a combination of NIPPV with PEEP followed by high-flow nasal cannula (HFNC) O_2 for presaturation during UEI. This study is in progress. This technique holds promise to attenuate hypoxemia by combining 2 techniques for presaturation in patients at high risk of desaturation during UEI. These studies have been performed by groups that favor RSI where some period of apnea occurs around the time of endotracheal tube insertion. The utility of HFNC and NIPPV with GSI, where a patient may continue to breathe spontaneously during endotracheal tube insertion, has not been formally investigated. Intuitively, these preoxygenation methods might be particularly effective with GSI, because patients might entrain the O_2 flow more efficiently than during apnea.

GASTRIC ULTRASONOGRAPHY

Aspiration of gastric contents is uncommon in elective operating room endotracheal intubation, because it is a uniform standard that patients be nothing by mouth before any planned operation. Because this is not possible in the emergency situation, an occasional complication of UEI is massive aspiration of gastric contents. Patients with a full stomach may vomit during UEI due to laryngeal stimulation and/or gastric air insufflation, resulting in a large volume of fluid entering the airway of the supine patient with reduced airway protective reflexes. One means of reducing this risk is by identifying the presence of gastric fluid before induction, and, based on its identification, to take action to reduce risk of its aspiration. Ultrasonography is well suited to identify fluid within the stomach because gastric fluid has distinctive characteristics on ultrasonography examination, appearing as a relatively hypoechoic space surrounded by typical anatomic boundaries. Two methods have been described:

1. The probe is placed over the lower lateral left thorax in the mid to posterior axillary line with the tomographic plane in coronal axis. The spleen is identified and used as a sonographic window to identify the stomach and any consequential collection of fluid within it.[26]
2. The probe is placed over the anterior epigastric region with the tomographic plane in sagittal axis. The examiner angles the probe side-to-side to identify the stomach and any potentially consequential collection within it.[27] One limitation to the anterior approach is that air within the stomach may block visualization of fluid that has collected in a dependent location.

If a significant fluid collection is present, the team may choose to insert a nasogastric tube to empty the stomach. If a patient is too unstable to tolerate nasogastric tube insertion, 2 suction devices are set up with team members specifically assigned to their immediate use should the need arise. The most experienced team member is assigned to insert the endotracheal tube.

The skilled operator can perform ultrasonography examination for gastric fluid in a short period of time while the team is setting up other required equipment for UEI. The authors recommend that the critical care team consider incorporating gastric ultrasonography into their standard checklist approach to UEI.

IMPROVING THE SAFETY OF URGENT ENDOTRACHEAL INTUBATION

A systematic approach to preintubation assessment, mobilization of equipment and personnel, and standardization of patient preparation prior to UEI could mitigate the morbidity and mortality associated with UEI. Mosier and colleagues[28] showed that implementation of an 11-month simulation-based curriculum emphasizing recognition and preparedness for the difficult airway improved first-pass success rate from 74% to 84% in the post-training period. Back-up plans for failed intubation attempts and immediate postintubation management were emphasized in simulation scenarios.

Use of a goal-directed, team-based approach to organize equipment and to keep clinicians focused, has been shown to be effective. Jaber and colleagues[29] showed that implementation of a bundled intubation protocol with 10 checklist items was associated with a significant decrease in life threatening complications. Mayo and colleagues[10] reported an iterative process to improve overall safety of UEI. The project used didactic training, task training, and deliberate practice using simulation-based training with a computerized patient simulator combined with crew resource management tactics; postevent briefings to prepare pulmonary, critical care, and sleep medicine fellows to deal with real-life UEI scenarios; and a mandatory multi-item do/confirm checklist.

SUMMARY

1. UEI is associated with a variety of dangerous complications
2. The number of attempts and time required to perform endotracheal intubation is a common metric used to assess quality of critical care airway management; a more sophisticated analysis focuses on the maintenance of physiologic function.
3. The MACOCHA score is useful as a predictor of difficult airway.
4. RSI and GSI are both effective means of induction during endotracheal intubation.
5. Both DL and VL are effective means to guide endotracheal intubation. Operators with limited training in DL may consider VL a primary tool.
6. Effective preoxygenation is an important element to reduce risk of severe desaturation during UEI.
7. Gastric ultrasonography is a useful method for identification of gastric fluid.
8. Focused training in critical care airway management may reduce complication rate of UEI.

REFERENCES

1. Jaber S, Amraoui J, Lefrant JY, et al. Clinical practice and risk factors for immediate complications of endotracheal intubation in the intensive care unit: a prospective, multiple-center study. Crit Care Med 2006;34:2355–61.
2. De Jong A, Molinari N, Terzi N, et al. Early identification of patients at risk for difficult intubation in the intensive care unit: development and validation of the MACOCHA score in a multicenter cohort study. Am J Respir Crit Care Med 2013;187:832–9.
3. Mosier JM, Joshi R, Hypes C, et al. The physiologically difficult airway. West J Emerg Med 2015;16:1109–17.
4. Kerslake D, Oglesby AJ, Di Rollo N, et al. Tracheal intubation in an urban emergency department in Scotland: a prospective, observational study of 3738 intubations. Resuscitation 2015;89:20–4.
5. Buis ML, Maissan IM, Hoeks SE, et al. Defining the learning curve for endotracheal intubation using direct laryngoscopy: a systematic review. Resuscitation 2016;99:66–71.
6. Bernhard M, Mohr S, Weigand MA, et al. Developing the skill of endotracheal intubation: implication for emergency medicine. Acta Anaesthesiol Scand 2012;56:164–71.

7. Barjaktarevic I, Berlin D. Bronchoscopic intubation during continuous nasal positive pressure ventilation in the treatment of hypoxemic respiratory failure. J Intensive Care Med 2015;30:161–6.

8. Koenig SJ, Lakticova V, Narasimhan M, et al. Safety of propofol as an induction agent for urgent endotracheal intubation in the medical intensive care unit. J Intensive Care Med 2015;30:499–504.

9. Lakticova V, Koenig SJ, Narasimhan M, et al. Video laryngoscopy is associated with increased first pass success and decreased rate of esophageal intubations during urgent endotracheal intubation in a medical intensive care unit when compared to direct laryngoscopy. J Intensive Care Med 2015;30:44–8.

10. Mayo PH, Hedge A, Eisen LA, et al. A program to improve the quality of emergency endotracheal intubation. J Intensive Care Med 2011;26:50–6.

11. Lewis SR, Butler AR, Parker J, et al. Videolaryngoscopy versus direct laryngoscopy for adult patients requiring tracheal intubation [review]. Br J Anaesth 2017;119:369–83.

12. De Jong A, Molinari N, Conseil M, et al. Video laryngoscopy versus direct laryngoscopy for orotracheal intubation in the intensive care unit: a systematic review and meta-analysis. Intensive Care Med 2014;40:629–39.

13. Huang HB, Peng JM, Xu B, et al. Video laygngoscopy for endotracheal intubation of critically ill adults: a systemic review and meta-analysis. Chest 2017;152: 510–7.

14. Mosier JM, Whitmore SP, Bloom JW, et al. Video laryngoscopy improves intubation success and reduces esophageal intubations compared to direct laryngoscopy in the medical intensive care unit. Crit Care 2013;17:237–45.

15. Kory P, Guevarra K, Mathew JP, et al. The impact of video laryngoscopy use during urgent endotracheal intubations in the critically ill. Anesth Analg 2013;117: 144–9.

16. Silverberg MJ, Li N, Acquah SO, et al. Comparison of video laryngoscopy versus direct laryngoscopy during urgent endotracheal intubation: a randomized controlled trial. Crit Care Med 2015;43:636–41.

17. Lascarrou JB, Boisrame-Helms J, Bailly A, et al. Video laryngoscopy vs direct laryngoscopy on successful first-pass orotracheal intubation among ICU patients: a randomized clinical trial. JAMA 2017;317:483–93.

18. Ambrosio A, Pfannenstiel T, Bach K, et al. Difficult airway management for novice physicians: a randomized trial comparing direct and video-assisted laryngoscopy. Otolaryngol Head Neck Surg 2014;150:775–8.

19. Mort TC. Preoxygenation in critically ill patients requiring emergency tracheal intubation. Crit Care Med 2005;33:2672–5.

20. Mort TC, Waberski BH, Clive J. Extending the preoxygenation period from 4 to 8 mins in critically ill patients undergoing emergency intubation. Crit Care Med 2009;37:68–71.

21. Baillard C, Fosse JP, Sebbane M, et al. Noninvasive ventilation improves preoxygenation before intubation of hypoxic patients. Am J Respir Crit Care Med 2006;174:171–7.

22. Sakles JC, Mosier JM, Patanwala AE, et al. First pass success without hypoxemia is increased with the use of apneic oxygenation during rapid sequence intubation in the emergency department. Acad Emerg Med 2016;23:703–10.

23. Miguel-Montanes R, Hajage D, Messika J, et al. Use of high-flow nasal cannula oxygen therapy to prevent desaturation during tracheal intubation of intensive care patients with mild-to-moderate hypoxemia. Crit Care Med 2015;43:574–83.

24. Vourc'h M, Asfar P, Volteau C, et al. High-flow nasal cannula oxygen during endotracheal intubation in hypoxemic patients: a randomized controlled clinical trial. Intensive Care Med 2015;41:1538–48.
25. Jaber S, Monnin M, Girard M, et al. Apnoeic oxygenation via high-flow nasal cannula oxygen combined with non-invasive ventilation preoxygenation for intubation in hypoxaemic patients in the intensive care unit: the single-centre, blinded, randomised controlled OPTINIV trial. Intensive Care Med 2016;2:1877–87.
26. Koenig SJ, Lakticova V, Mayo PH. Utility of ultrasonography for detection of gastric fluid during urgent endotracheal intubation. Intensive Care Med 2011;37:627–31.
27. Hamada SR, Garcon P, Ronot M, et al. Ultrasound assessment of gastric volume in critically ill patients. Intensive Care Med 2014;40:965–72.
28. Mosier JM, Malo J, Sakles JC, et al. The impact of a comprehensive airway management training program for pulmonary and critical care medicine fellows. A three-year experience. Ann Am Thorac Soc 2015;12:539–48.
29. Jaber S, Jung B, Corne P, et al. An intervention to decrease complications related to endotracheal intubation in the intensive care unit: a prospective, multiple-center study. Intensive Care Med 2010;36:248–55.

Asynchrony Consequences and Management

Tài Pham, MD, PhD[a,b], Irene Telias, MD[a,b], Thomas Piraino, RRT[c],
Takeshi Yoshida, MD, PhD[a,b,d], Laurent J. Brochard, MD[a,b,*]

KEYWORDS

- Mechanical ventilation • Dyssynchrony • Airway pressure • Monitoring
- Work of breathing

KEY POINTS

- Dyssynchrony is a mismatch between the patients' inspiratory and expiratory times and the mechanical ventilator delivery.
- Dyssynchrony is associated with worse outcomes, but causality has not been shown; it is unknown if controlling dyssynchrony can lead to a better outcome.
- There is not a single dyssynchrony, but several types with different mechanisms, consequences, and potential management.
- A simple visual monitoring of the ventilator screen can detect gross dyssynchrony, but automated systems are needed.

INTRODUCTION: WHAT IS DYSSYNCHRONY AND WHY DOES IT MATTER?

Mechanical ventilation is the most common life support procedure in the intensive care unit (ICU).[1] It is used in a full spectrum of acute situations, which share the same primary goals: to maintain gas exchange, reduce the work of breathing, and improve patient comfort. Depending on the severity and timing of the patients' course, mechanical ventilation can fully control and suppress the patients' respiratory load or be used as partial ventilatory support, that is, preserving spontaneous effort to a certain extent. An ideal delivery of mechanical ventilation would reduce respiratory distress by decreasing excessive respiratory load, while maintaining an appropriate level of spontaneous effort (preventing diaphragm and respiratory muscle atrophy)

[a] Interdepartmental Division of Critical Care Medicine, University of Toronto, St. Michael's Hospital, 30 Bond Street, Toronto, ON M5B 1W8, Canada; [b] Keenan Research Centre for Biomedical Science, Li Ka Shing Knowledge Institute, St. Michael's Hospital, 209 Victoria Street, Toronto, ON M5B 1T8, Canada; [c] Department of Respiratory Therapy, St. Michael's Hospital, 30 Bond Street, Toronto, ON M5B 1W8, Canada; [d] Translational Medicine, Departments of Critical Care Medicine and Anesthesia, Hospital for Sick Children, University of Toronto, 555 University Avenue, Toronto, ON M5G 1X8, Canada
* Corresponding author. Keenan Research Centre for Biomedical Science, Li Ka Shing Knowledge Institute, St. Michael's Hospital, 209 Victoria Street, Toronto, ON M5B 1T8, Canada.
E-mail address: BrochardL@smh.ca

Crit Care Clin 34 (2018) 325–341
https://doi.org/10.1016/j.ccc.2018.03.008
0749-0704/18/© 2018 Elsevier Inc. All rights reserved.

with harmonious patient-ventilator interaction. However, this situation is not always met; when this fragile balance is jeopardized, patient-ventilator dyssynchrony occurs. Dyssynchrony is defined as a mismatch between the patients' own inspiratory and expiratory times and the mechanical ventilator delivery.[2] This mismatch often reveals a discrepancy between the patients' needs and the amount of assistance delivered by the machine. Dyssynchrony then becomes a complex phenomenon involving interaction of the ventilator with several organs, namely, the lungs; the respiratory muscles, including the diaphragm; and the nervous system, including the respiratory centers[3] (**Fig. 1**). Dyssynchrony detection requires a careful examination of flow and airway pressure (Paw) waveforms displayed on the ventilator screen,[4] along with clinical examination of the patients' breathing pattern. Dyssynchronies can easily be missed by clinicians who cannot continuously stare at the screen or may not recognize them. More advanced monitoring, for example, using esophageal manometry or electrical activity of the diaphragm, can help clinicians to detect dyssynchrony; but these are not routinely used in daily clinical practice.[5,6]

Ventilated patients are regularly managed while ignoring dyssynchrony: so why should we focus on this topic? *First*, even if precise epidemiologic data on dyssynchrony are lacking, it seems to be a frequent event in ventilated patients; we can roughly estimate that at least one-third of patients exhibit frequent dyssynchrony during mechanical ventilation.[7-10] *Second*, observational studies have consistently found dyssynchrony to be associated with poor outcomes, such as longer duration of ventilatory support and higher mortality.[8,11] Reducing dyssynchrony by adapting ventilatory conditions is often feasible.[12,13] Therefore, although association does not prove causality, there might be a chance to improve clinical outcomes by reducing/avoiding patient-ventilator dyssynchrony. Dyssynchrony may contribute to lung injury or respiratory muscle dysfunction as well as having an impact on patient comfort.

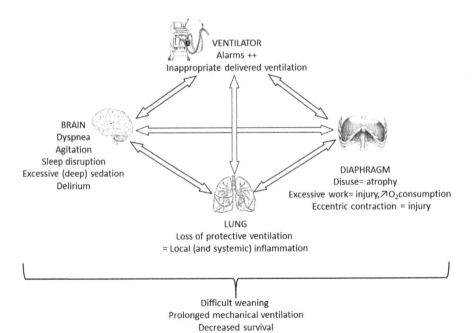

Fig. 1. Interactions between organs and ventilator involved in dyssynchrony and their consequences.

In this review, the authors define the different types of dyssynchrony and then consider the evidence for their association with patient outcomes and discuss their potential management. Remaining uncertainties and areas for improvement are also examined. For clarity and didactic reasons, only dyssynchrony in adult patients during invasive mechanical ventilation will be considered, keeping the pediatric population and noninvasive ventilation out of the scope of this review.

DYSSYNCHRONY: DEFINITIONS AND MECHANISTIC CLASSIFICATION

Dyssynchronies are often classified based on the phase of the respiratory cycle: trigger phase, pressurization (inspiratory phase), and cycling off to the expiratory phase.[14,15] This classification facilitates diagnosis at the bedside using the available waveforms.[4] However, an approach centered on the condition that led to the mismatch may help to understand the underlying mechanism and to design a treatment strategy.

Derangements of respiratory drive and inspiratory effort often occur in patients with acute respiratory failure under mechanical ventilation. The control of breathing under mechanical ventilation becomes complex and includes feedback signals from central and peripheral chemoreceptors as well as mechanoreceptors and vagal inputs from the lung, chest wall, and respiratory muscles.[16] Additional stimuli, such as pain, anxiety, or endotoxemia, can directly influence respiratory centers. A high respiratory drive can result from increased metabolic demands but also in the context of altered gas exchange and/or intense mechanical stimuli through lung receptors.[17] On the other hand, a low respiratory drive is due to either a primarily depressed central nervous system, often by (excessive) sedation, and/or an excessive ventilatory support.[16] Patient-ventilator dyssynchronies occur primarily in the context of either high respiratory drive (usually associated with insufficient assistance) or low respiratory drive (usually related to overassistance).

High Respiratory Drive (Insufficient Assistance)

Flow starvation

Flow starvation occurs when gas delivery does not fully meet the patients' ventilatory demand. It can be recognized on the Paw tracing[4] as a concave indentation as if patients were sucking or pulling air from the ventilator proportionally to the increased muscular pressure (**Fig. 2**A). Although the ventilator is still helping inflation to some degree, the result is an additional imposed load to patients and an increased energy expenditure of the respiratory muscles.[18] This phenomenon is typically present during volume assist control, when the ventilator targets a preset peak flow (with either a square wave or decelerating pattern) that does not completely meet the patients' needs. Marini and colleagues[19] were the first to describe relative flow starvation and to raise the importance of correctly setting inspiratory flow during assist-control ventilation.

Short (or premature) cycling: double triggering/breath-stacking

Short cycling occurs when patients' inspiratory effort continues during the mechanical expiration (**Fig. 2**B). Activation of inspiratory muscles during mechanical deflation (lengthening) results in an eccentric contraction of the diaphragm,[20] which is potentially injurious for the respiratory muscles. When strong enough, it can trigger a second mechanical breath (double triggering) before complete exhalation of the first one, resulting in an increased total tidal volume. This latter phenomenon is also named breath-stacking,[21] because of the occurrence of a new breath on top of the previous one. Breath-stacking is frequent in patients with acute respiratory

A

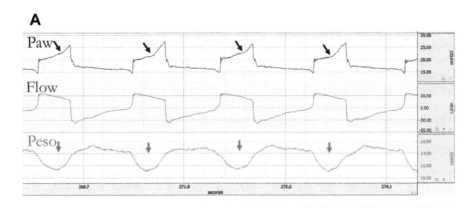

B

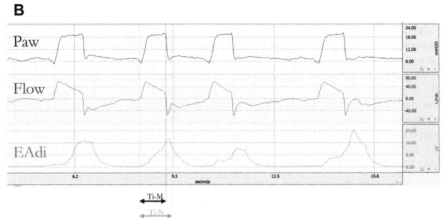

Fig. 2. (*A*) Example of a tracing with relative flow starvation: the ventilator is in a volume assist-control mode with decelerating flow. The flow delivered by the ventilator does not meet the patient's need. During the inspiration phase, there is a concave deflection of the Paw (*blue arrow*), whereas the Peso shows a negative deflection indicating patient's effort (*green arrow*). (*B*) Example of short cycling in a pressure support ventilation. The patient's neural inspiration time (Ti-N from triggering to the moment EAdi decrease to 70% of the maximal EAdi) is longer than the actual breath delivered by the ventilator (Ti-M). EAdi, electrical activity of the diaphragm; Peso, esophageal pressure; Ti-M, machine insufflation time; Ti-N, neural inspiration time.

failure during low tidal volume ventilation.[22] In a group of patients with early moderate to severe acute respiratory distress syndrome (ARDS) without neuromuscular blocking agents, an average of 27 breath-stacking events occurred per hour in the first 72 hours following intubation, with an average peak number of events of 170 per hour.[21] Moreover, double triggering was the second most common dyssynchrony in a heterogeneous population of spontaneously breathing patients under mechanical ventilation in a study by Thille and colleagues[8]; an association between double triggering, lower Pao_2/fraction of inspired oxygen (Fio_2) ratio, and higher peak inspiratory pressures was observed. This finding, together with a higher respiratory rate in these patients, suggests that this type of asynchrony occurs more frequently in patients with worse lung injury and increased respiratory drive. Several ventilator factors contribute to this type of asynchrony: an inverse association between double triggering and set tidal volume[22]; being ventilated with assist-control ventilation[8]; and having a shorter set inspiratory time, including during pressure support ventilation (PSV).[23]

The obvious consequence of breath-stacking is the delivery of high tidal volume and lung stress. The tidal volume delivered during these events was 1.6[22] and 1.8[21] times higher than the preset tidal volume in 2 different studies using low tidal volume ventilation, reaching 10.1 mL/kg and 11.3 mL/kg of predicted body weight (PBW), respectively.

Low Respiratory Drive (Overassistance)

Reverse triggering resulting in ineffective effort or double cycling

In cases of deep sedation and decreased respiratory drive, mechanical insufflation generated by the ventilator can trigger a muscular effort. Akoumianaki and colleagues[24] first described this type of asynchrony, named reverse triggering, in acutely ill patients under mechanical ventilation.[24] It occurs during controlled mechanical ventilation. The first breath is triggered by the ventilator and is followed by inspiratory activity of the respiratory muscles. If esophageal pressure (Peso) or electrical activity of the diaphragm (EAdi) is being used for monitoring, a decrease in Peso or an increase in EAdi after the beginning of mechanical insufflation is diagnostic of reverse triggering (**Fig. 3**A). In the absence of these monitoring tools, an increase in expiratory flow or decrease in inspiratory Paw later in the respiratory cycle can indicate the event. Additionally, if the inspiratory effort is strong enough, a second breath can be delivered by the ventilator, resulting in breath-stacking, as described earlier for high respiratory drive (**Fig. 3**B). The difference with double triggering induced by a high drive is that the first breath in the case of reverse triggering is a mandatory breath (not triggered by patients). It is probably a frequent phenomenon, being present in all the patients of a small cohort of consecutive, heavily sedated patients with ARDS under mechanical ventilation.[24] Deep sedation suppresses the cortical influence on respiratory drive, allowing this phenomenon to occur, or at least, to be identified.

The precise mechanism is unknown but somehow related to respiratory entrainment described in healthy humans[25,26] and animals.[27] The term *entrainment* refers to the fixed, repetitive, temporal relationship between mechanical insufflation and neural inspiration, requiring afferent input from the lungs and/or chest wall. Initially thought to be mediated through vagal afferents, the phenomenon was found in patients after lung transplant[26] suggesting that vagal inputs are not required. Additionally, it was described in brain-dead patients,[28] raising the possibility of mechanoreceptors in muscles and chest wall, local spinal reflexes, or a more complex spinal respiratory pattern generator to be involved in the process.

Interestingly, consequences of reverse triggering are probably the same as the ones of short cycling and double triggering during high respiratory drive: lengthening contractions of the diaphragm and breath-stacking with increased tidal volume.[8,21,22]

Delayed cycling

Delayed cycling occurs when mechanical insufflation continues after neural inspiration has ceased or even during active expiration. It can be detected by comparing mechanical insufflation with the duration of inspiratory effort using Peso or EAdi[4] (**Fig. 4**A).

During PSV, the ventilator cycles to expiration when flow decreases to a set percentage of peak inspiratory flow. Insufflation tends to be longer with higher levels of pressure support and with increased airflow resistance. Additionally, higher levels of pressure support result in a higher peak flow that may shorten neural inspiratory time,[29] further contributing to a mismatch between a long mechanical insufflation

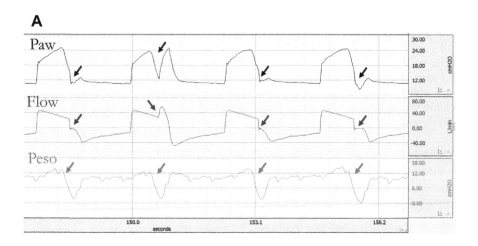

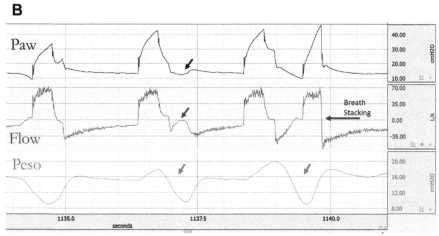

Fig. 3. (A) Example of reverse triggering in volume assist-control with decelerating flow. Each insufflation is time triggered (machine controlled); in the middle (breath 2) or at the end of the inspiration phase (breaths 1, 3, and 4), a negative deflection of the Peso occurs (reverse triggering, *green arrow*) leading to a negative deflection of the Paw (*blue arrow*) and increasing flow during the machine insufflation phase or slowing it during the machine expiratory phase (*pink arrows*). (B) Example of reverse triggering and breath-stacking in volume assist-control. The first breath is patient triggered, the second is machine triggered and followed by a reverse triggering (*first green arrow*) starting in the late phase of machine insufflation and continuing during the early phase of machine exsufflation (leading to a positive deflection of the flow [*pink arrow*] not triggering a new breath); the third breath is machine triggered, followed by a reverse triggering (*second green arrow*). This reverse triggering leads to a fourth breath before complete exhalation of the previous one (breath-stacking). EAdi, electrical activity of the diaphragm; Ti-M, machine insufflation time; Ti-N, neural inspiration time.

and a short neural inspiratory time. Patients with chronic obstructive pulmonary disease (COPD) and asthma are at particular risk, and the shorter expiratory time contributes to worsening hyperinflation in these patients.[30] Moreover, overassistance results in hyperventilation, hypocapnia, respiratory alkalosis, reducing respiratory drive, and perpetuating the mechanism.

A

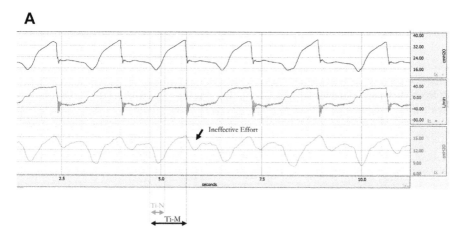

B

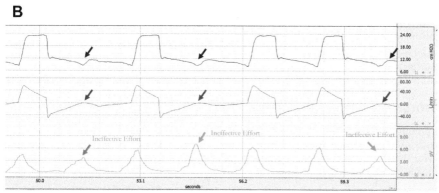

Fig. 4. (*A*) Example of delayed cycling (followed by ineffective efforts) in volume assist-control. The breath delivered by the ventilator (Ti-M) is longer than the actual patient's effort (Ti-N from the start of the effort to the moment Peso decrease to 70% of the maximal Peso deflection). Each breath delivered by the ventilator is followed by an ineffective effort in the early phase of the machine exsufflation. (*B*) Example of a tracing with ineffective efforts: The ventilator is in PSV mode. Three patient's efforts (*green arrows*) are not triggering a machine insufflation. At the time of the wasted effort, a positive deflection in the airway flow tracing (*pink arrow*) and a negative deflection in the Paw (*blue arrow*) can be noticed. Ti-M, machine insufflation time; Ti-N, neural inspiration time.

Ineffective efforts

Ineffective effort is the most frequent type of dyssynchrony in patients under invasive mechanical ventilation, both early in the course of the disease and during prolonged mechanical ventilation.[7–9,11] Clinical evidence of inspiratory effort not followed by mechanical insufflation is specific for the diagnosis,[7] but probably not very sensitive. Contrary to circumstances associated with high drive, patients frequently look calm and not dyspneic.[31] A decrease in Paw tracing concurrent with an increase in flow during expiration is suggestive, and a negative deflection in Peso or significant increase in EAdi not followed by a mechanical breath is diagnostic[4] (**Fig. 4**B). Delayed cycling and overassistance are the two main causes, especially in the presence of airflow obstruction: this leads to hyperinflation and intrinsic positive end-expiratory pressure PEEP (PEEPi).[12,32,33] Additionally, overassistance contributes to decrease respiratory drive.[12,34] The patients' effort starts before the end of exhalation and becomes insufficient to overcome PEEPi, resulting in failure to trigger a mechanical breath.[33] Decreased respiratory drive by other mechanisms, such as sedation, increases the occurrence of ineffective efforts.[9] Deeper levels of sedation with propofol have been associated with lower respiratory drive and higher frequency of ineffective efforts during PSV.[35] Ineffective efforts result in wasted energy expenditure of the respiratory muscles. The inspiratory effort in such circumstances often does not change with lower levels of assistance but without wasted efforts.[7,12,34] Ineffective efforts during expiration are likely lengthening (or eccentric) contractions of the diaphragm, with the potential for muscle injury. They also often indicate excessive levels of ventilation.

Central apneas during sleep
Through hyperventilation, PSV can cause central apnea associated with sleep disruption in healthy subjects[36] and in patients under invasive mechanical ventilation[37]: when $Paco_2$ decreases to less than a certain threshold, an apnea event may occur. Apneas are more frequent during sleep because the $Paco_2$ threshold triggering apnea is higher during sleep than during wakefulness and more easily reached. Apnea, with or without desaturation, rapidly results in sleep disruption (arousal or awakening) and sleep fragmentation making it impossible to reach deep sleep stages.

The apnea will often trigger an alarm on the ventilator and may switch the ventilator to a rescue mode.[36] This mechanism of apnea is exacerbated in patients with heart failure[37] that have a longer circulation time and increased chemoreceptive sensitivity.

ASSOCIATION WITH POOR OUTCOME

Accumulating evidence suggests that patient-ventilator dyssynchrony is associated with poor outcomes, including higher mortality and longer durations of ventilation and ICU stay.[7,8,11,38,39] Although association is not a synonym of causality, a strong physiologic rationale could explain these observations. In patients with a high respiratory drive, flow starvation and breath-staking with increased tidal volume could lead to the clinical failure of lung protective ventilation (resulting in a worse outcome) and also in respiratory muscle injury.

Dyssynchronous breathing has been shown to produce episodic increases in transpulmonary pressure, potentially leading to ventilation-associated lung injury (VALI).[40] Animal models have shown that spontaneous breathing can worsen lung injury, especially in severe ARDS models.[41] Suppression of these types of breaths is a potentially important means of limiting VALI. This suppression could be an explanation for the reduction of mortality and duration of mechanical ventilation found in patients with ARDS and a Pao_2/Fio_2 ratio less than 150 mm Hg receiving neuromuscular blockade, by fully suppressing respiratory efforts and dyssynchrony.[42]

More than 20 years ago, Chao and colleagues[7] showed that ineffective efforts were associated with increased duration of mechanical ventilation and a lower rate of weaning success. Their population was somewhat specific, including only ventilator-dependent patients referred to their specialized unit, but their assessment of ineffective effort was accurate and confirmed by esophageal catheter in a subgroup of patients. A few other studies focusing on the relationship between dyssynchrony and outcomes had 2 frequent limitations: a short period of ventilation was assessed[8,38] and/or all types of dyssynchrony were considered together.[8,11,43] The study results are summarized in **Table 1**. In 2006, Thille and colleagues[8] confirmed the link between the rate of dyssynchrony and outcomes. In invasively ventilated patients awake and starting to trigger the ventilator (in assist control ventilation or PSV modes), they recorded 30 minute periods of flow and Paw signals. Patients with a

Table 1
Main cohort studies looking at dyssynchrony

Author, Year	Chao et al,[7] 1997	Thille et al,[8] 2006	Pohlman et al,[22] 2008	de Wit et al,[38] 2009	Blanch et al,[11] 2015	Beitler et al,[21] 2016	Vaporidi et al,[39] 2017
Type of dyssynchrony	Ineffective efforts	Ineffective efforts Double-triggering Auto-triggering Short cycle Prolonged cycle	Double triggering	Ineffective efforts	Ineffective efforts Double-triggering Aborted Inspiration Short cycle Prolonged cycle Auto-triggering	Double-triggering	Ineffective efforts
Population	Prolonged MV	As soon as patients triggered breaths	ALI and low tidal volume	First 24 h, Pao₂ Fio₂ ratio >150, PEEP ≤10	Expected to be ventilated for >24 h	ARDS first 24 h in assist control	Controlled ventilation >12 h
N of patients	174	62	20	60	50	33	110
Mode MV	VCV/AC	VCV/AC, PSV		VCV/AC or PCV/AC SIMV + PSV, PSV	VCV/AC or PCV/AC, PSV	VCV/AC	PSV and PAV
Hours of MV		31	23		7027	1841	2931
Recording duration	>2 min	30 min	5 d	10 min	≈80% of total duration of MV	72 h	24 h
N Breaths				11,482	8,731,981	2 millions	4,456,537

(continued on next page)

Table 1
(continued)

Author, Year	Chao et al,[7] 1997	Thille et al,[8] 2006	Pohlman et al,[22] 2008	de Wit et al,[38] 2009	Blanch et al,[11] 2015	Beitler et al,[21] 2016	Vaporidi et al,[39] 2017
Prevalence	11% had IE AI = 45 ± 13.8%	24% had AI >10% AI = 2.1% DT = 13% IE = 85%	Mean: 2.3 ± 3.5 DT per minute DT: 9.7% of breaths	27% had AI >10%	Median AI = 3.41% (IQR = 1.95–5.77)	DT = 27 breaths/h Hourly peak = 170 breaths/h At least one DT during 72% of hours recorded	AI = 2.43 [IQR 1.1–5.1] 12% had AI >10% 30.4% had clusters IE
Risk factors	IE: COPD, Higher age, higher $Paco_2$, lower MIP	DT: More sedated patients; Lower Pao_2 Fio_2 ratio; VCV/AC mode; shorter Ti; higher PEEP IE: Male gender; COPD; higher bicarbonates; alkalosis; higher PS and PIP; less sensitive trigger; higher VT	DT: Lower set VT	AI >10%: Pressure triggered breath and higher intrinsic respiratory rate	DT more frequent in PCV/AC and PSV IE: more frequent in PSV and with higher PS		Clusters of IE: more frequent in patients with sepsis
Outcome	IE associated with lower rate of weaning success (16% vs 57%)	AI >10% associated with longer MV and higher rate of tracheostomy		IE associated with longer duration of MV, longer ICU and Hospital stay	AI >10% associated with higher ICU and hospital mortality		Clusters of IE in the 1st recording associated with longer duration of MV and higher mortality

Abbreviations: AI, asynchrony index; ALI, acute lung injury; ARDS, acute respiratory distress syndrome; COPD, chronic obstructive pulmonary disease; DT, double triggering; Fio_2, inspired oxygen fraction; ICU, intensive care unit; IE, ineffective efforts; IQR, interquartile range; MIP, maximal inspiratory pressure; MV, mechanical ventilation; $Paco_2$, arterial partial pressure of carbon dioxide; Pao_2, arterial partial pressure of oxygen; PAV, proportional-assist ventilation; PCV/AC, pressure assist-control ventilation; PEEP, positive end-expiratory pressure; PIP, peak inspiratory pressure; PS, pressure support; PSV, pressure support ventilation; SIMV, synchronized intermittent mandatory ventilation; Ti, inspiratory time; VCV/AC, volume assist-control ventilation; VT, tidal volume.

dyssynchrony index (ratio defined by the number of dyssynchronous breath over the total number of breath including ineffective efforts) higher than 10% had a longer duration of mechanical ventilation and a higher rate of tracheostomy. Obtaining recordings early in the course of mechanical ventilation and focusing only on ineffective efforts, de Wit and colleagues[38] found similar results using multivariable analysis: patients with a dyssynchrony index of 10% or greater had a longer duration of mechanical ventilation, ICU and hospital stay, and were less likely to be discharged home. The development of automatized techniques[44] made the analysis of longer recordings feasible and not limited by the time to visually review recordings. Blanch and colleagues[11] continuously recorded airflow and Paw in 50 patients from intubation to liberation from the ventilator or death and demonstrated that a dyssynchrony index greater than 10% was associated with higher ICU and hospital mortality. More recently, Vaporidi and colleagues[39] focused on the time variation of dyssynchrony and elegantly introduced the concept of clusters of dyssynchrony. Only taking into account ineffective efforts, they defined a cluster as periods of time containing more than 30 dyssynchronies in a 3-minute period. They performed 24-hour recordings on intubated patients as soon as they were receiving PSV or proportional-assist ventilation (PAV). In the 110 patients analyzed, they found that clusters of dyssynchrony, and not the dyssynchrony index, were associated with a longer duration of mechanical ventilation and higher hospital mortality. The only discordant study that did not find an association between dyssynchrony and outcome is an ancillary analysis of a study comparing PSV with neurally adjusted ventilator assist (NAVA) for liberation from mechanical ventilation. Patients were included when they could tolerate PSV for at least 30 minutes; Paw and flow as well as EAdi were recorded for 20-minute sessions at 12, 24, 36, and 48 hours following inclusion. Determining the dyssynchrony index by visual assessment using EAdi, they found that 83% of the patients had a dyssynchrony index greater than 10% and it was not associated with outcomes. Interestingly, repeating the analysis only using flow and pressure waveforms without EAdi found a very different rate of patients with a dyssynchrony index greater than 10% (7% vs 83%) raising the question of the specificity and sensitivity of each method and the definition of dyssynchronies.

MANAGEMENT

Just as cardiac dysrhythmia, all types of dyssynchrony are not identical. Dyssynchronies may result from different mechanisms, have different consequences and impact on clinical outcomes. Some may require active management, whereas some may be passive bystanders that could simply be ignored. The authors currently lack evidence to recommend which dyssynchrony should precisely be treated and which should be tolerated.

Several risk factors have been described for different types of dyssynchrony suggesting that controlling these factors could decrease dyssynchrony and proposed management for their reduction (see **Table 1** and below). Although neuromuscular blocking agents abolish all types of dyssynchrony, like in severe ARDS, it is not a reasonable option for all types of dyssynchrony. Ineffective effort and breath-stacking are the 2 types of dyssynchrony that have been the most extensively studied.

Ineffective Efforts

Ventilatory settings
Ineffective efforts occur when the patients' effort is not strong enough to reach a certain trigger threshold. A way to facilitate triggering is to increase the trigger sensitivity to make the threshold easier to attain or to switch from a pressure to a flow trigger,[45] but this is often not sufficient. Most of the time it is caused by ventilator

overassistance, decreased respiratory drive, and intrinsic PEEP that patients cannot overcome to trigger the breath.[34] In a cohort of patients with COPD tested with different levels of PS and PEEP, Nava and colleagues[32] found that the application of an external PEEP of 75% of the intrinsic PEEP was efficient to reduce the work of breathing and ineffective efforts, as later confirmed by Chao and colleagues[7] in their population with prolonged ventilation. Thille and colleagues[12] systematically tested ventilator setting optimization in patients on PSV with an ineffective triggering index greater than 10%; they assessed 2 different levels of PEEP (0 vs 5 cm H_2O) and then the effect of PS reduction by steps of 2 cm H_2O or reducing insufflation time by increasing the cycling-off by steps of 10%. They showed that the most effective way to decrease ineffective efforts was to reduce overassistance by decreasing pressure support: they were completely eliminated in two-thirds of the patients. Optimizing inspiratory time allowing smaller tidal volume was also an efficient way to decrease ineffective efforts.[46]

Proportional modes of ventilation

Proportional modes of ventilation have been shown to decrease patient-ventilator dyssynchrony.[47–51] During NAVA[52] and PAV,[53] the ventilator generates pressure in proportion to the patients' instantaneous effort.[54] Therefore, these modes usually avoid overassistance[55]; gas delivery follows the patients' breathing pattern in terms of amplitude and timing much better than classic modes like PSV. The cycling mechanism is based on the end of the flow signal in PAV and on a decrease of EAdi to 75% of the peak with NAVA. The triggering is optimized with NAVA, using the EAdi signal directly. In addition, in response to an increased load, patients receive higher ventilatory support, resulting in lower inspiratory effort per minute compared with PSV.[56,57]

Proportional-assist ventilation

During PAV, the muscular effort is estimated noninvasively by the ventilator, based on measured flow, Paw, elastance, and resistance. The proportion of ventilator assistance relative to the patients' muscular effort is defined by the clinician as a percentage.

Giannouli and colleagues[58] proved that at high levels of support, tidal volume is higher with PSV and there are, consequently, more ineffective efforts compared with PAV. Others confirmed that patients on PAV have less ineffective efforts and other asynchronies compared with PSV.[47,50,59] The clinical consequences remain to be determined.

The avoidance of overassistance should result in less central apnea events during sleep. In fact, Bosma and colleagues[47] showed that patients on PAV had less arousals, awakenings, and more rapid eye movement and slow wave sleep than on PSV. The number of arousals per hour was correlated with asynchronies and respiratory muscle unloading. In contrast, Alexopoulou and colleagues,[50] despite proving the lower number of asynchronies with PAV compared with PSV, did not find less sleep fragmentation on PAV. This finding could have been related to the design of the study, patients spending less time on each mode for one night, or to the type of patients because PAV may not work as efficiently when there is substantial intrinsic PEEP (COPD).

Neurally adjusted ventilatory assist

NAVA requires the insertion of a special nasogastric tube with an array of electrodes that sense EAdi. Clinicians set the NAVA level, which determines the amount of pressure delivered per unit of EAdi. The ventilator is triggered and cycled off by the EAdi signal.[52]

Several physiologic studies[35,60–63] showed a frank reduction in the number of asynchronies in patients under NAVA compared with PSV. Interestingly, given the trigger criteria, there are virtually no ineffective efforts during NAVA.[35,61,62] Cycling from inspiration to expiration occurs when the EAdi signal reaches 70% of the peak. In patients with low respiratory compliance and high drive, premature cycling and double triggering can still be present.[63]

Breath-Stacking

Breath-stacking is a concerning consequence of dyssynchrony (short cycling or reverse triggering) that can hinder protective ventilation and induce lung injury. It is a source of VALI by delivering tidal volume up to twice the set volume. Breath-stacking seems frequent in patients with a high respiratory drive.[21,22] In a cohort of patients with ARDS with continuous recording of flow and Paw, Pohlman and colleagues[22] found a mean frequency of 2.3 stacked breaths per minute (accounting for 9.7% of the breaths) leading to a median volume of stacked breath of 10.1 mL/kg PBW (when tidal volumes were set at 5.9 mL/kg PBW). No intervention was performed to reduce the occurrence of breath-stacking, but they found in a multivariable analysis that lower set tidal volume was the only factor associated with this dyssynchrony. In another cohort of 66 intubated patients presenting breath-stacking in more than 10% of breaths, Chanques and colleagues[13] showed that modifying ventilator settings decreased the median breath-stacking index from 38% to 2%. To a lesser extent, increasing sedation reduced this index from 41% to 27%. In a multivariable analysis, switching from an assisted control mode to PSV and increasing inspiratory time in assist control ventilation were the 2 factors associated with breath-stacking decrease. Last, but not least, neuromuscular blocking agents totally abolish breath-stacking[21] allowing to completely control patients' ventilation.[42]

SUMMARY

Dyssynchrony is a frequent and polymorphic event during the entire course of invasive mechanical ventilation, with high interindividual and intraindividual variability. Different types of dyssynchrony have different physiologic causes and consequences and also require different management. Current knowledge on dyssynchrony mainly comes from small physiologic or observational studies, and precise epidemiologic data are lacking. Many questions related to dyssynchrony assessment and management remain unanswered: are short periods of monitoring enough or should continuous assessment be the rule? Are airway and pressure waveforms sufficient or should monitoring of respiratory muscle activity (esophageal catheter or EAdi) be systematically used? Is the association with outcome confounded by severity or an actual causal link? Which types of dyssynchronies are harmful? Finally, would intervention aiming at reducing dyssynchrony improve patient outcomes? Dyssynchrony is far from revealing all its secrets.

ACKNOWLEDGMENTS

The authors thank Felipe Damiani and Ricard Mellado Artigas for their help in reviewing examples of waveforms displaying dyssynchrony.

REFERENCES

1. Mehta AB, Syeda SN, Wiener RS, et al. Epidemiological trends in invasive mechanical ventilation in the United States: a population-based study. J Crit Care 2015;30:1217–21.
2. Mauri T, Yoshida T, Bellani G, et al, PLeUral pressure working Group (PLUG— acute respiratory failure section of the European Society of intensive care

medicine). Esophageal and transpulmonary pressure in the clinical setting: meaning, usefulness and perspectives. Intensive Care Med 2016;42:1360–73.

3. Blanch L, Quintel M. Lung-brain cross talk in the critically ill. Intensive Care Med 2017;43:557–9.

4. Georgopoulos D, Prinianakis G, Kondili E. Bedside waveforms interpretation as a tool to identify patient-ventilator asynchronies. Intensive Care Med 2006;32: 34–47.

5. Bellani G, Laffey JG, Pham T, et al, LUNG SAFE Investigators, ESICM Trials Group. Epidemiology, patterns of care, and mortality for patients with acute respiratory distress syndrome in intensive care units in 50 countries. JAMA 2016; 315:788–800.

6. Duan EH, Adhikari NKJ, D'Aragon F, et al. Management of acute respiratory distress syndrome and refractory hypoxemia. A multicenter observational study. Ann Am Thorac Soc 2017;14:1818–26.

7. Chao DC, Scheinhorn DJ, Stearn-Hassenpflug M. Patient-ventilator trigger asynchrony in prolonged mechanical ventilation. Chest 1997;112:1592–9.

8. Thille AW, Rodriguez P, Cabello B, et al. Patient-ventilator asynchrony during assisted mechanical ventilation. Intensive Care Med 2006;32:1515–22.

9. de Wit M, Pedram S, Best AM, et al. Observational study of patient-ventilator asynchrony and relationship to sedation level. J Crit Care 2009;24:74–80.

10. Colombo D, Cammarota G, Alemani M, et al. Efficacy of ventilator waveforms observation in detecting patient-ventilator asynchrony. Crit Care Med 2011;39: 2452–7.

11. Blanch L, Villagra A, Sales B, et al. Asynchronies during mechanical ventilation are associated with mortality. Intensive Care Med 2015;41:633–41.

12. Thille AW, Cabello B, Galia F, et al. Reduction of patient-ventilator asynchrony by reducing tidal volume during pressure-support ventilation. Intensive Care Med 2008;34:1477–86.

13. Chanques G, Kress JP, Pohlman A, et al. Impact of ventilator adjustment and sedation-analgesia practices on severe asynchrony in patients ventilated in assist-control mode. Crit Care Med 2013;41:2177–87.

14. Gilstrap D, MacIntyre N. Patient-ventilator interactions. Implications for clinical management. Am J Respir Crit Care Med 2013;188:1058–68.

15. Tobin MJ, Jubran A, Laghi F. Patient-ventilator interaction. Am J Respir Crit Care Med 2001;163:1059–63.

16. Georgopoulos D, Roussos C. Control of breathing in mechanically ventilated patients. Eur Respir J 1996;9:2151–60.

17. Brochard L, Slutsky A, Pesenti A. Mechanical ventilation to minimize progression of lung injury in acute respiratory failure. Am J Respir Crit Care Med 2017;195: 438–42.

18. MacIntyre NR, McConnell R, Cheng KC, et al. Patient-ventilator flow dyssynchrony: flow-limited versus pressure-limited breaths. Crit Care Med 1997;25: 1671–7.

19. Marini JJ, Capps JS, Culver BH. The inspiratory work of breathing during assisted mechanical ventilation. Chest 1985;87:612–8.

20. Gea J, Zhu E, Gáldiz JB, et al. Functional consequences of eccentric contractions of the diaphragm. Arch Bronconeumol 2009;45:68–74.

21. Beitler JR, Sands SA, Loring SH, et al. Quantifying unintended exposure to high tidal volumes from breath stacking dyssynchrony in ARDS: the BREATHE criteria. Intensive Care Med 2016;42:1427–36.

22. Pohlman MC, McCallister KE, Schweickert WD, et al. Excessive tidal volume from breath stacking during lung-protective ventilation for acute lung injury. Crit Care Med 2008;36:3019–23.
23. Tokioka H, Tanaka T, Ishizu T, et al. The effect of breath termination criterion on breathing patterns and the work of breathing during pressure support ventilation. Anesth Analg 2001;92:161–5.
24. Akoumianaki E, Lyazidi A, Rey N, et al. Mechanical ventilation-induced reverse-triggered breaths: a frequently unrecognized form of neuromechanical coupling. Chest 2013;143:927–38.
25. Graves C, Glass L, Laporta D, et al. Respiratory phase locking during mechanical ventilation in anesthetized human subjects. Am J Physiol 1986;250:R902–9.
26. Simon PM, Habel AM, Daubenspeck JA, et al. Vagal feedback in the entrainment of respiration to mechanical ventilation in sleeping humans. J Appl Physiol (1985) 2000;89:760–9.
27. Muzzin S, Baconnier P, Benchetrit G. Entrainment of respiratory rhythm by periodic lung inflation: effect of airflow rate and duration. Am J Physiol 1992;263:R292–300.
28. Delisle S, Charbonney E, Albert M, et al. Patient-ventilator asynchrony due to reverse triggering occurring in brain-dead patients: clinical implications and physiological meaning. Am J Respir Crit Care Med 2016;194:1166–8.
29. Fernandez R, Mendez M, Younes M. Effect of ventilator flow rate on respiratory timing in normal humans. Am J Respir Crit Care Med 1999;159:710–9.
30. Chiumello D, Polli F, Tallarini F, et al. Effect of different cycling-off criteria and positive end-expiratory pressure during pressure support ventilation in patients with chronic obstructive pulmonary disease. Crit Care Med 2007;35:2547–52.
31. Schmidt M, Banzett RB, Raux M, et al. Unrecognized suffering in the ICU: addressing dyspnea in mechanically ventilated patients. Intensive Care Med 2014;40:1–10.
32. Nava S, Bruschi C, Rubini F, et al. Respiratory response and inspiratory effort during pressure support ventilation in COPD patients. Intensive Care Med 1995;21:871–9.
33. Parthasarathy S, Jubran A, Tobin MJ. Cycling of inspiratory and expiratory muscle groups with the ventilator in airflow limitation. Am J Respir Crit Care Med 1998;158:1471–8.
34. Leung P, Jubran A, Tobin MJ. Comparison of assisted ventilator modes on triggering, patient effort, and dyspnea. Am J Respir Crit Care Med 1997;155:1940–8.
35. Vaschetto R, Cammarota G, Colombo D, et al. Effects of propofol on patient-ventilator synchrony and interaction during pressure support ventilation and neurally adjusted ventilatory assist. Crit Care Med 2014;42:74–82.
36. Meza S, Mendez M, Ostrowski M, et al. Susceptibility to periodic breathing with assisted ventilation during sleep in normal subjects. J Appl Physiol (1985) 1998;85:1929–40.
37. Parthasarathy S, Tobin MJ. Effect of ventilator mode on sleep quality in critically ill patients. Am J Respir Crit Care Med 2002;166:1423–9.
38. de Wit M, Miller KB, Green DA, et al. Ineffective triggering predicts increased duration of mechanical ventilation. Crit Care Med 2009;37:2740–5.
39. Vaporidi K, Babalis D, Chytas A, et al. Clusters of ineffective efforts during mechanical ventilation: impact on outcome. Intensive Care Med 2017;43:184–91.
40. Yoshida T, Fujino Y, Amato MBP, et al. Fifty years of research in ARDS. Spontaneous breathing during mechanical ventilation. Risks, mechanisms, and management. Am J Respir Crit Care Med 2017;195:985–92.

41. Yoshida T, Uchiyama A, Matsuura N, et al. The comparison of spontaneous breathing and muscle paralysis in two different severities of experimental lung injury. Crit Care Med 2013;41:536–45.

42. Papazian L, Forel J-M, Gacouin A, et al, ACURASYS Study Investigators. Neuromuscular blockers in early acute respiratory distress syndrome. N Engl J Med 2010;363:1107–16.

43. Rolland-Debord C, Bureau C, Poitou T, et al. Prevalence and prognosis impact of patient-ventilator asynchrony in early phase of weaning according to two detection methods. Anesthesiology 2017;127(6):989–97.

44. Blanch L, Sales B, Montanya J, et al. Validation of the Better Care® system to detect ineffective efforts during expiration in mechanically ventilated patients: a pilot study. Intensive Care Med 2012;38:772–80.

45. Aslanian P, El Atrous S, Isabey D, et al. Effects of flow triggering on breathing effort during partial ventilatory support. Am J Respir Crit Care Med 1998;157: 135–43.

46. Tassaux D, Gainnier M, Battisti A, et al. Impact of expiratory trigger setting on delayed cycling and inspiratory muscle workload. Am J Respir Crit Care Med 2005; 172:1283–9.

47. Bosma K, Ferreyra G, Ambrogio C, et al. Patient-ventilator interaction and sleep in mechanically ventilated patients: pressure support versus proportional assist ventilation. Crit Care Med 2007;35:1048–54.

48. Terzi N, Pelieu I, Guittet L, et al. Neurally adjusted ventilatory assist in patients recovering spontaneous breathing after acute respiratory distress syndrome: physiological evaluation. Crit Care Med 2010;38:1830–7.

49. Costa R, Spinazzola G, Cipriani F, et al. A physiologic comparison of proportional assist ventilation with load-adjustable gain factors (PAV+) versus pressure support ventilation (PSV). Intensive Care Med 2011;37:1494–500.

50. Alexopoulou C, Kondili E, Plataki M, et al. Patient-ventilator synchrony and sleep quality with proportional assist and pressure support ventilation. Intensive Care Med 2013;39:1040–7.

51. Schmidt M, Kindler F, Cecchini J, et al. Neurally adjusted ventilatory assist and proportional assist ventilation both improve patient-ventilator interaction. Crit Care 2015;19:56.

52. Sinderby C, Navalesi P, Beck J, et al. Neural control of mechanical ventilation in respiratory failure. Nat Med 1999;5:1433–6.

53. Younes M. Proportional assist ventilation, a new approach to ventilatory support. Theory. Am Rev Respir Dis 1992;145:114–20.

54. Lellouche F, Brochard L. Advanced closed loops during mechanical ventilation (PAV, NAVA, ASV, SmartCare). Best Pract Res Clin Anaesthesiol 2009;23:81–93.

55. Kacmarek RM. Proportional assist ventilation and neurally adjusted ventilatory assist. Respir Care 2011;56:140–8 [discussion: 149–52].

56. Ranieri VM, Giuliani R, Mascia L, et al. Patient-ventilator interaction during acute hypercapnia: pressure-support vs. proportional-assist ventilation. J Appl Physiol (1985) 1996;81:426–36.

57. Grasso S, Puntillo F, Mascia L, et al. Compensation for increase in respiratory workload during mechanical ventilation. Pressure-support versus proportional-assist ventilation. Am J Respir Crit Care Med 2000;161:819–26.

58. Giannouli E, Webster K, Roberts D, et al. Response of ventilator-dependent patients to different levels of pressure support and proportional assist. Am J Respir Crit Care Med 1999;159:1716–25.

59. Xirouchaki N, Kondili E, Vaporidi K, et al. Proportional assist ventilation with load-adjustable gain factors in critically ill patients: comparison with pressure support. Intensive Care Med 2008;34:2026–34.
60. Colombo D, Cammarota G, Bergamaschi V, et al. Physiologic response to varying levels of pressure support and neurally adjusted ventilatory assist in patients with acute respiratory failure. Intensive Care Med 2008;34:2010–8.
61. Spahija J, de Marchie M, Albert M, et al. Patient-ventilator interaction during pressure support ventilation and neurally adjusted ventilatory assist. Crit Care Med 2010;38:518–26.
62. Piquilloud L, Vignaux L, Bialais E, et al. Neurally adjusted ventilatory assist improves patient-ventilator interaction. Intensive Care Med 2011;37:263–71.
63. Mauri T, Bellani G, Grasselli G, et al. Patient-ventilator interaction in ARDS patients with extremely low compliance undergoing ECMO: a novel approach based on diaphragm electrical activity. Intensive Care Med 2013;39:282–91.

Determinants and Prevention of Ventilator-Induced Lung Injury

Francesco Vasques, MD, Eleonora Duscio, MD,
Francesco Cipulli, MD, Federica Romitti, MD, Michael Quintel, MD,
Luciano Gattinoni, MD*

KEYWORDS

- Mechanical ventilation • Ventilator-induced lung injury
- High-volume and high-pressure ventilation • Acute respiratory distress syndrome
- Mechanical power

KEY POINTS

- Mechanical ventilation has adverse side effects.
- Ventilatior-induced lung injury results from the interaction between the lung parenchyma and the mechanical forces applied on it.
- High PEEP may favor barotrauma, while lower PEEP may favor atelectrauma. Risks and benefits of PEEP in a range between 5 to 15 cm H_2O are equivalent, while at higher PEEP the risks of volutrauma outweight the benefits of reduces atelectrauma.

INTRODUCTION

As every powerful treatment, mechanical ventilation has its adverse side effects, which are classically referred to as ventilator-induced lung injury (VILI) and were first recognized—mainly as gross barotrauma—soon after the introduction of mechanical ventilation in patients with acute respiratory distress syndrome (ARDS). In the 1960s, the goal of mechanical ventilation was to maintain a normal gas exchange. The effort to limit the increase in CO_2 in patients with severely impaired lung compliance and increased dead space was obtained through high-volume and high-pressure ventilation, which often led to pneumothorax. This complication was so frequent that some authors suggested the preemptive positioning of chest drain in patients with ARDS.[1–3] Nowadays, this scenario seems to be hardly believable, but it must be pointed out that, back in the 1970s, the most feared complications of mechanical ventilation

Department of Anesthesiology, Emergency and Intensive Care Medicine, University of Göttingen, Robert-Koch-Straße 40, Göttingen 35075, Germany
* Corresponding author. Department of Anesthesiology, Emergency and Intensive Care Medicine, University of Göttingen, Robert-Koch-Straße 40, Göttingen 37075, Germany.
E-mail address: gattinoniluciano@gmail.com

Crit Care Clin 34 (2018) 343–356
https://doi.org/10.1016/j.ccc.2018.03.004
0749-0704/18/© 2018 Elsevier Inc. All rights reserved.

were those related to a high fraction of inspired oxygen. It has been forgotten, but the first applications of extracorporeal support were designed to reduce the fraction of inspired oxygen in patients with ARDS, and certainly not to allow less mechanically aggressive ventilation.[4] For years, therefore, barotrauma was considered an easily treatable complication (ie, drainage) and an unavoidable price to pay for keeping the patient alive. The remarkable conceptual change, however, was introduced by Dreyfuss and colleagues,[5] who emphasized the importance of volume—instead of airway pressure—in determining the ventilation-related lung damage. Actually, strictly speaking, volume and pressure are the 2 faces of the same coin, because they are linked by a proportionality constant: the total elastance of the respiratory system (ie, the sum of the chest wall and lung elastance). In cases of increased chest wall elastance, for the same high-pressure ventilation, lung damage was not observed, because most of the pressure was spent to displace the thorax instead of distending the lung. Obviously, the differences between volutrauma and barotrauma vanish when considering the *lung's* transpulmonary pressure and changes in *lung* volume. In an era in which the transpulmonary pressure was just a physiologic issue—remote from whatever clinical application—the concept of volutrauma represented an intellectual advance and pointed out that the lung lesions were due to excessive strain (ie, "movement" is required to promote damage). The concept of volutrauma paralleled the progressive attention to the decrease in tidal volume, first implemented in asthmatic patients. Hickling and colleagues[6] introduced the same concept of "permissive hypercapnia" as a tool for more gentle treatment of the ARDS lung. The landmark National Institutes of Health randomized trial documented the worse outcome of high tidal volume compared with the lower one. The next step toward a better understanding of the relationship between mechanical ventilation and lung damage was due to Slutsky's group in Toronto who, in an ex vivo rat lung model, showed that the damage resulting from mechanical ventilation was in large part due to the cyclic opening and closing of lung units, preventable by applying adequate positive end-expiratory pressure (PEEP).[7] This experiment was in line with the previous theoretic consideration of Mead and associates[8] and Lachmann,[9] and further reinforced by the clinical work of Amato and coworkers[10] and Ranieri and colleagues.[11] Indeed, Slutsky's experiments helped open the way to a new concept: to keep the lung open with PEEP may not only make mechanical ventilation safer, it might even promote lung recovery. In the last years, consequently, the effort to reduce mechanical ventilation-related lung damages converted into the widespread acceptance of the open lung strategy (ie, high PEEP associated with a low tidal volume) as the best way for treating patients with ARDS. However, several banks of clinical data seem to contrast with this belief. Therefore, despite decades of experimental and clinical research, which we briefly summarized, several issues remain open: (1) The definition and the assessment of VILI in the clinical setting seem, per se, to be questionable; (2) What is the mortality attributable to VILI in mechanically ventilated patients?; (3) Which are actual mechanical triggers of VILI?; and finally (4) Which are the lung conditions that favor it? Only when we will have answered these questions, we will be able to formulate a rational and, most likely, a predictably effective approach to VILI prevention.

DEFINITION OF VENTILATOR-INDUCED LUNG INJURY

The acronym VILI may express 2 concepts: *ventilator*-induced lung injury, stressing the importance of the ventilatory setting, or *ventilation*-induced lung injury, in which the emphasis is on the consequences of the forces acting on lung parenchyma during either spontaneous or mechanical ventilation. Indeed—regardless the origin of the force (ie, spontaneous or mechanical)[12]—for a given condition, the damages will be roughly equivalent if we neglect the hemodynamic drawbacks, which are different during mechanical ventilation (blood pushed out of the thorax) or during spontaneous breathing (blood pulled into the thorax). Owing to the vagueness of this definition, it is not surprising that VILI includes a wide series of lung damages, ranging from edema to gross pneumothorax. Indeed, depending on the putative cause of lung damage addressed by the different authors, over the years VILI has been further defined as barotrauma, volutrauma, atelectrauma, or biotrauma. Although VILI mechanisms have been intensively investigated in several experimental models, its "diagnosis" and quantification in ARDS is elusive, because its manifestations are indistinguishable from ARDS itself. It is even possible that VILI is an unavoidable component of ARDS that cannot exist without mechanical ventilation (ie, life-saving treatment). In a sense, we could say that VILI—to an undetermined extent—is part of the natural history of ARDS.

THE NATURE OF VENTILATOR-INDUCED LUNG INJURY

In line with a recent series of experiments, we postulate that VILI is caused by the delivery of a critical amount of mechanical energy to the lung. The word critical could refer to:

1. An amount of energy determining a structural deformation sufficient to activate mechanotransduction-related inflammation or create microwounding.
2. Mechanical energy sufficient to break molecular bonds of the fibers composing the extracellular matrix.[3] The resulting polymers may activate the inflammatory reaction through a stimulation of toll receptors.

It is important, however, to emphasize 1 concept: the mechanical energy is either so great as to cause stress-at-rupture (eg, pneumothorax) or, when below the stress-at-rupture threshold, it is delivered for a sufficient time. In other words, the greater the mechanical energy applied over time, the greater the amount of lung damage (ie, microfractures) in the extracellular matrix and the cell membrane. Above a certain, unknown threshold of energy/time, the rate of microscopic damage will eventually overcome the repair capability of the lung structures, leading to VILI. Therefore, energy and time are the 2 essential components of VILI development and, considered together, they define the mechanical power.

The Mechanical Power

Indeed, all mechanical factors implied in ventilation—namely, tidal volume, driving pressure, flow, resistances, respiratory rate, and PEEP—are different components of a unique physical variable, which is the energy delivered over time, that is, the mechanical power. Strictly speaking, the mechanical power should be expressed in watts (ie, joule/s). However, this represents the intensity of the mechanical ventilation, whereas VILI—below stress at rupture—depends greatly on the duration of energy application. Therefore, we prefer to express the mechanical power in joules per minute.

The mechanical power is derived by multiplying each component of the motion equation by the tidal volume.[13] Accordingly, in the respiratory system we have:

$$Power_{rs} = 0.098 \cdot RR \cdot \left\{ \Delta V^2 \cdot \left[\frac{1}{2} \cdot E_{rs} + RR \cdot \frac{(1+I:E)}{60 \cdot I:E} \cdot R_{aw} \right] + \Delta V \cdot PEEP \right\} \qquad (1)$$

Where 0.098 is the conversion factor from L/cm H_2O to Joules; RR is the respiratory rate, ΔV is the tidal volume, E_{RS} is the elastance of the respiratory system; I:E is the ratio between inspiratory and expiratory time; and R_{aw} are the airway resistances. The term $E_{RS}\frac{1}{2}\Delta V^2$ is the energy required to inflate the respiratory system (ie, dynamic power when related to time; the $E_{RS}\Delta V$ product equals the driving pressure). The term $\Delta V^2 \cdot RR \cdot \frac{(1+I:E)}{60 \cdot I:E} \cdot R_{aw}$ is the energy required to overcome the airways and tissue resistances (ie, the resistive power, when related to time). The term $\Delta V \cdot PEEP$ is the energy required to equilibrate the potential energy stored in the system at PEEP level (ie, "static" power when related to time).

The mechanical power applied to the lung was computed as follows:

$$Power_L = 0.098 \cdot RR \cdot \Delta V^2 \cdot \left(\frac{1}{2}E_L + \text{Lung resistances}\right) + \Delta V \cdot [(Paw_{PEEP} - Paw_{ZEEP})$$
$$- (Pes_{PEEP} - Pes_{ZEEP})]$$

(2)

Where E_L is the lung elastance; Paw_{PEEP} and Paw_{ZEEP} are the airway pressures measured at PEEP and Zero-end expiratory pressure (ZEEP), respectively; Pes_{PEEP} and Pes_{ZEEP} are the esophageal pressures measured at PEEP and ZEEP, respectively. Dynamic, resistive and static lung power mirror the components described above for the whole respiratory system.

It is possible to mathematically simplify the equation[1] as follows:

$$Power_{rs} = 0.098 \cdot RR \cdot \Delta V \cdot \left(P_{peak} - \frac{1}{2} \Delta P_{aw}\right)$$

(3)

Although the relative weight of each mechanical power component may vary in the different ventilatory settings, there is no doubt that its dynamic element plays a major role. Indeed, using mathematical exponents, the mechanical power is function of the tidal volume raised to the power of 2, the respiratory rate raised to the power of 1.4 and PEEP raised to the power of 1. It is, therefore, useful to analyze in some detail which are the relevant pressures and volumes through which VILI may occur. A wise management of mechanical ventilation should include the measurements discussed herein.

Delivery of Mechanical Power and Lung Inhomogeneity

When discussing how the delivery of mechanical energy can be injurious to the lung, we should address a spatial and a temporal factor, inquiring where the energy is distributed and during which phase of the respiratory cycle.

Spatial factor

The distribution pattern of the energy applied to the lung mainly depends on the homogeneity of the lung and it is mirrored by the distribution of strain and stress, which are direct consequences of energy application. Considering a homogeneous, theoretic system, each pulmonary unit receives the same quantum of energy, which is, therefore, evenly distributed (**Fig. 1**, left). Even the normal lung, however, is an inhomogeneous system, particularly where structures with different elasticity interface each other (eg, connection of fiber network to the visceral pleura). Furthermore, during pathologic processes, inhomogeneity can greatly increase, especially at the interface between collapsed and open pulmonary units (see **Fig. 1**, right). Indeed, a classical paper of by Mead and associates[8]—who studied stress and strain distribution between completely distended and completely collapsed units—suggested that, at the interface between normal and pathologic tissue, there is a focused stress considerably

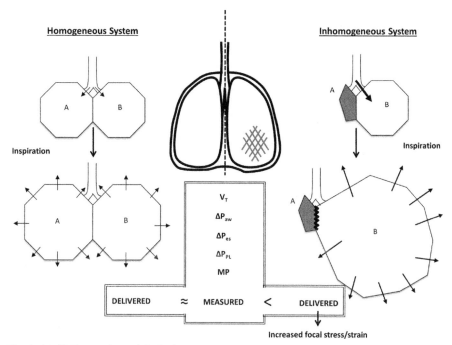

Fig. 1. (*Left*) Theoretic model of a homogeneous system, represented as 2 normal and identical pulmonary units. (*Right*) Theoretic model of an inhomogeneous system, represented as one atelectatic unit (*gray*) and a normal, contiguous unit (*white*). ΔP_{aw}, airway driving pressure; ΔP_{es}, driving esophageal pressure; ΔP_{pl}, driving transpulmonary pressure; MP, mechanical power; V_t, tidal volume.

greater than the average applied to the fully open lung. Mead computed that—at the interface between a unit inflated at its total capacity (volume = 10 arbitrary units) and 1 completely collapsed (volume = 1)—the focal stress would be equal to the stress applied to the lung times $10^{2/3}$ (a stress multiplier equal to 4.6). More recently, using computed tomography (CT) scan measurement of inhomogeneity, we estimated that the focal stress would increase by a factor of 2,[14] implying that a transpulmonary pressure of 30 cm H_2O would locally correspond with about 60 cm H_2O. Therefore, locally, the stress may be twice as great as the transpulmonary pressure applied to the whole lung. The associated energy, however, would be 4 times greater, because it increases with the square of the applied pressure.[13]

Temporal factor
Regarding the distribution of energy through the respiratory cycle, data are extremely scarce.[15] However, theoretic considerations suggest that the "damaging" energy may primarily be the one dissipated in the airways and in the lung tissue recoil during expiration. A model of this phenomenon is presented in **Fig. 2**.

THE ASSESSMENT OF VENTILATOR-INDUCED LUNG INJURY
Experimental Models

The assessment of lung edema is probably the most common method used to describe VILI in experimental models. Indeed, edema often manifests with the deterioration of lung mechanics and gas exchange, and it can be better quantified by lung

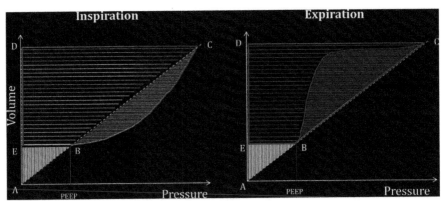

Fig. 2. (*Left*) Baseline energy (*red hatched triangle* ABE), on which the inspiratory energy associated with the tidal volume (area BCDE) is added. The *yellow hatched area* to the right of line BC represents the inspiratory dissipated energy needed to move the gas, to overcome surface tension forces, to make the extracellular sheets slide across one another (tissue resistances), and possibly to reinflate collapsed pulmonary units. The *light green hatched area* on the left of line BC defines the elastic energy (trapezoid EBCD) cyclically added to the respiratory system during inspiration. The total area included in the triangle ACD is the total energy level present in the respiratory system at end inspiration. (*Right*) Energy changes during expiration. Of the total energy accumulated at end inspiration (triangle ACD), the area of the trapezoid EBCD is the energy released during expiration. The fraction of energy included in the hysteresis area (*light blue hatched area*) is dissipated into the respiratory system, whereas the remaining area (*dark blue hatched area*) is energy dissipated into the atmosphere through the connecting circuit. Note that whatever maneuver (as controlled expiration) reduces the hysteresis area will reduce the energy dissipated into the respiratory system (potentially dangerous?). PEEP, positive end-expiratory pressure.

weight measured at the end of the experiment. Histology was largely used to detect further signs of lung damage, such as inflammatory infiltrates, septal rupture, or dilatation, as well as hemorrhage and emphysema. Circulating inflammatory mediators were also used, both as VILI indicators and as indirect estimate of capillary permeability. Finally, the quantitative CT scan analysis allows measurement of the lung weight and lung inhomogeneities. It is worth recalling, however, that VILI encompasses a wide range of different lesions, depending on the model and the mechanical ventilation setting used to induce VILI. As an example, VILI induced just by high-volume/high-pressure mechanical ventilation may have a different appearance depending on several variables, such as the degree of pressure used, the presence of PEEP, and its level. Different species may also react differently to similar insults[16] and time to injury plays a crucial role, as well. This is not the place for reviewing in detail the experimental literature on VILI; herein it is enough to clearly state that the prevalent damage may shift from mostly edema in model without PEEP (where atelectrauma may play a primary role) to models of high PEEP and high pressures, where the increased intrathoracic and alveolar pressures dampen edema formation, but accentuate hemodynamic impairment and volutrauma.

Clinical Practice

Regardless of the damage observed in animal experiments, it is worth noting that we do not have any direct method to really detect VILI during treatment of patients with ARDS. Whatever lesion due to VILI, in fact, is indistinguishable from the lesions present in ARDS independently of mechanical ventilation. We may even wonder, in this sense, if VILI would not be an unavoidable consequence of ARDS. Even without externally applied pressures, increased spontaneous breathing effort may induce injury. Inflammation induces capillary leakage and specific hyperventilation (VE/functional residual capacity [FRC]—baby lung) is always present in ARDS unless artificial lungs are applied. Indeed, it is important to realize that what we call experimental VILI is nothing else but the induction of experimental ARDS. Having said that, there is no doubt that unwise mechanical ventilation may aggravate the pattern of ARDS. The best proof we have is the ARDS trial on tidal volume, showing the risk in full-blown ARDS of using tidal volume causing 100% strain difference (12 mL/kg vs 6 mL/kg).[17] Therefore, we must understand that the assessment of what we call VILI in humans has only been tested by the outcome difference (ie, mortality). It is surprising, sometimes, to realize that most of the approaches to assess VILI in experimental animals are not even considered when dealing with VILI in the human being. In addition, we do not have a convincing idea about the precise relationship between VILI and mortality. In fact, mortality may occur days after mechanical ventilation has been withdrawn, changed, or modified. We do not understand how it is possible (if it is indeed possible), that a few hours of mechanical ventilation—for example, during anesthesia—might produce significant complications that manifest days afterward, even in normal patients. The VILI–outcome link in humans is missing.

VENTILATOR-INDUCED LUNG INJURY IN CLINICAL PRACTICE
What Is the Mortality Attributable to Ventilator-Induced Lung Injury

In the last 50 years, several ventilatory strategies have been introduced in the treatment of patients with ARDS, in whom the risk of VILI is remarkably higher than in other patients in the intensive care unit. Such approaches range from "protective" low-pressure and low-volume mechanical ventilation to the open lung approach and from high-frequency ventilatory oscillation to the extracorporeal CO_2 removal. As noted, in clinical trials efficacy in VILI prevention has mainly been evaluated as mortality reduction. Currently, the most accepted strategy consists in the use of low tidal volume with an undefined PEEP level (ie, protective lung approach). It is unknown, however, what is the mortality per se attributable to mechanical ventilation in ARDS. As an example, would a further reduction in tidal volume be beneficial? If yes, what is the expected benefit and in which patients may we observe it? In our opinion, the estimate of the attributable mortality should be the logical premise of any meaningful randomized trial, because its feasibility depends on this starting point. To illustrate, if the absolute attributable mortality is set at 6% of the actual mortality, to prove that a new treatment may reduce it to 0 (6% absolute decrease), in an ARDS population with a baseline mortality of 40%, the number of patients required (ie, the sample size) would be of 2030 patients (alpha 0.05, beta 0.2). Considering an enrollment rate of 0.3 patients per unit per month as usually observed in ARDS randomized, controlled trials, it follows that, to show a positive benefit, a study with 50 participating units would be accomplished in 11 years. In contrast, some investigators—to make the trial feasible—reduce the sample size by targeting an unrealistic decrease in mortality as high as 20% (EOLIA trial; NCT01470703). In this case, the trial will completed in less than one-half of the time, but the failure to reach the statistical significance is very likely. Unfortunately, this may lead to discarding potentially useful strategies.

Which Are the Conditions that Favor Ventilator-Induced Lung Injury?

As discussed, with the exception of gross barotrauma, it is virtually impossible to assess VILI per se in ARDS, because ventilation undoubtedly contributes to its pathophysiologic progression. Indeed, if the ARDS lung is sufficiently small and inhomogeneous, mechanical ventilation or even spontaneous breathing are intrinsically contributing to its damage in the form of stress and strain. However, in the context of mild or mild to moderate ARDS—considering the available data and experience—it is possible to deliver relatively safe ventilation with acceptable mechanical power. Therefore, whatever attempt to reduce or abolish the risk of VILI needs a characterization of the patient's lungs (size and homogeneity) and a proper set of all ventilation components. This may be the only way to rationally estimate the risk of VILI for a given ventilatory setting.

Lung Size (Functional Residual Capacity)

It is easily understandable that the application of safe ventilation first requires the measurement of the aerated lung size (FRC). Indeed, the tidal volume per kilogram of predicted body weight represented an attempt to normalize the tidal volume to the lung size, assuming this to be proportionate to the predicted body weight. Unfortunately, this is not true in ARDS, where a 70-kg man, depending on ARDS severity, may have ventilatable lung size ranging from 300 mL up to 1500 mL. Although lung compliance and other mechanical variables are related to the lung size, this theoretic approximation is too weak to be reasonably applied to the individual patient. Therefore, ventilated lung size must be measured. There are several investigative methods to measure it, such as quantitative CT scan analysis or helium dilution.[18] A few ventilators recently introduced automatic FRC measurement by the gas dilution techniques. Surprisingly, the FRC measurement is largely ignored in clinical practice. This, however, does not decrease its fundamental importance in tailoring safe ventilation.

End-Expiratory Lung Volume

The end-expiratory lung volume (EELV) refers to the sum of FRC plus the volume owing to PEEP and, by definition, it coincides with FRC only in the absence of external or self-generated (auto) PEEP. Indeed, PEEP volume may be relevant. For example, in an individual with an FRC of 2000 mL and a respiratory system compliance of 100 mL/cm H_2O, 5 cm H_2O PEEP is roughly equivalent to a delta volume above the normal resting value of 500 mL, and 15 cm H_2O PEEP determines a delta volume about 3-fold greater (1500 mL), with an increase of about 75% FRC volume. The same percentage may apply to ARDS, because the specific compliance (ie, compliance/FRC) of the baby lung is similar to normal.[19] Therefore, 15 cm H_2O PEEP applied in a severe ARDS lung with an FRC of 500 mL would inflate the baby lung by 375 mL, almost doubling its unstressed volume. Of note, this phenomenon is partially independent from recruitability, as the recruited units—once open to gases—contribute minimally to the increase in gas volume.[14] The difference between the FRC and the EELV is relevant to better understand the concept of stress, strain, and why PEEP is a component of mechanical power. At FRC, strictly speaking, the lung is partially already stressed and strained, because the lung volume at FRC owing to negativity of the pleural pressure is distended compared with an isolated lung. It is convenient, however, to ignore this amount of strain and stress, assuming that at FRC stress and strain are equal to zero. When PEEP is applied to the respiratory system, the delta volume owing to PEEP corresponds with an increased end-expiratory transpulmonary pressure. This pressure produces a reactive force inside the fiber system—with the magnitude equal to the one applied and opposite direction—that, at end-expiration, is stored in the lung as potential energy. This force is called stress. Importantly, although equal in magnitude, stress is not the transpulmonary pressure, but it is the force developed in the structure that counterbalances the transpulmonary pressure. Accordingly, in ARDS, a PEEP level of 15 to 20 cm H_2O may generate already relevant stress and strain at end-expiration. From this condition, to inflate the lung an amount greater than the potential energy stored at EELV must be introduced in the system at each breath, therefore adding further stress and strain. In this framework, it is clear why strain should be computed relative to the FRC (excluding PEEP-related volume). Indeed, $\Delta V/EELV$ would produce an artificial decrease in computed strain, as the lung distortion is applied to a lung, which is already stressed by PEEP.

End-Inspiratory Lung Volume

This represents the sum of FRC, PEEP volume, and tidal volume, and is the maximal expansion imposed to the lung and end-inspiration. It is worth noting that the ratio between the end-inspiratory lung volume and total lung capacity, where total lung capacity is approximately 3 times FRC, has been found, in experimental work, to be of extreme importance. A ratio of 1 indicates that each breath reaches the physical limit of lung expansion, where all the collagen fibers are maximally extended. The application of strain exceeding that value in an experimental model led to VILI and death in 48 hours or less.

Atelectrauma Versus Volutrauma

In clinical practice, VILI is associated primarily with 2 phenomena: atelectrauma and volutrauma. These 2 conditions recognize 2 different mechanisms, whose prevention or correction are, unfortunately, opposite. Indeed, the ideal prevention of atelectrauma requires the use of very high volumes, and the prevention of volutrauma consists in avoiding such volumes. As shown in **Fig. 3**, atelectrauma and volutrauma lead to different consequences. Indeed, atelectrauma mainly consists in focal stress, whereas volutrauma is by definition an excessive, general stress and strain applied to the lung. Both injurious mechanisms are likely to produce microfractures in the lung matrix, activate local inflammation increasing capillary permeability, and, potentially, cause edema. Nonetheless, in experimental conditions, although edema is the most frequent finding in atelectrauma, it is usually a minor feature when volutrauma dominates, because high intrapulmonary volumes are determined by high pressures,

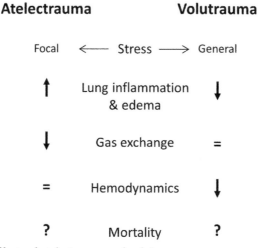

Fig. 3. The main effects of atelectrauma and volutrauma.

which prevent edema formation. Consequently, gas exchange is frequently near normal in pure atelectrauma, whereas it will progressively deteriorate when volutrauma-related edema develops. Despite the classical definition of VILI focuses on the lung only, the mechanical ventilation may deeply impact on the general hemodynamics, especially when high volumes/pressures are applied. Although these events are clearly defined in experimental models, their translation to ARDS is merely putative and assessed by comparing outcome during different modes of ventilation. The dilemma between atelectrauma and volutrauma, in principle, is the one that all the trials comparing higher and lower PEEP tried to resolve. Indeed, lower PEEP favors atelectrauma and should prevent volutrauma, whereas, in contrast, higher PEEP, will favor volutrauma by preventing atelectrauma. In a general ARDS population, the results of most of the studies so far performed indicate that the risk of barotrauma versus atelectrauma are equivalent in the range of pressures and volume applied. More specifically, 3 large studies compared higher versus lower PEEP (approximately cm H_2O 15 vs approximately 9 cm H_2O)[20–22] finding no difference in the outcome. This finding clearly suggests that, at this pressure level, the potential harms of atelectrauma are neither inferior nor superior to the potential harms of volutrauma. A more recent study, however, compared a little bit higher level of PEEP (approximately 16 cm H_2O), associated with a recruitment maneuver to lower PEEP ventilation (13 cm H_2O) without recruitment maneuvers.[23] The higher PEEP recruitment arm aimed at a greater prevention of atelectrauma than applied in the previous trials. Conversely, this strategy appeared harmful, as mortality was significantly higher in the higher PEEP recruitment patients (55.3% vs 49.3%; $P = .04$). This finding suggests that higher level of pressure than applied in the previous trials favors volutrauma, which is more harmful than atelectrauma. In addition, it is worth remembering that in normal clinical practice, the PEEP applied even in severe ARDS is usually set below 10 cm H_2O. A picture of the real-life ventilatory approach to patients with ARDS is provided by 3 observations studies, which included unselected patients with ARDS and, therefore, should adequately mirror clinical practice (**Table 1**).[24–26] For the sake of completeness, we added data retrieved from randomized, controlled trials who enrolled selected patients with ARDS.[17,20,22,23,27–30] As shown, in the observational studies the average level of PEEP was 8 to 9 cm H_2O—reaching values of 16 cm H_2O or higher only in randomized, controlled trials[23]—whereas plateau pressure was held at less than 30 cm H_2O. Although these data do not originate from randomized, controlled trials, they clearly suggest that, in the daily "battlefield" of ARDS treatment, the intensive care doctors consider the risk of volutrauma more dangerous than that of possible atelectrauma. A further piece of evidence on the hazard of high static pressures derives from 2 randomized, controlled trials comparing high-frequency ventilatory oscillation versus standard ventilation. Although 1 study found no outcome difference in the 2 groups,[31] Ferguson and colleagues[32] found a greater mortality in the high-frequency ventilatory oscillation patients. Indeed, this technique is characterized by lung volumes close to total lung capacity on which a remarkable amount of energy is imposed through the high-frequency oscillations.

HOW BEST TO PREVENT VENTILATOR-INDUCED LUNG INJURY

From what has been discussed herein, we think that the following suggestions should be considered to keep mechanical ventilation as safe as possible. We here refer only to patients in whom the respiratory system compliance is the range of 30 mL/cm H_2O and the Pao_2/fraction of inspired oxygen ratio is less than 150 mm Hg (ie, in patients

Table 1
Observational studies and clinical trials on acute respiratory distress syndrome

	Author, Year											
	Brochard et al,[27] 1998	Stewart et al,[28] 1998	Brower et al,[29] 1999	ARDSnet et al,[17] 2000	Esteban et al,[24] 2002	Brower et al,[22] 2004	Meade et al,[20] 2008	Briel et al,[34] 2010	Villar et al,[25] 2011	Guérin et al,[30] 2013	Bellani et al,[26] 2016	ART et al,[23] 2017
Type	RCT	RCT	RCT	RCT	Observational	RCT	RCT	Meta-analysis	Observational	RCT	Observational	RCT
No. of patients	58 58	60 60	100 100	387 405	231	236 258	508 475	1163 1136	255	229[a]	2377	500
V_t/PBW (mL/kg)	7.1 10.3	7.0 10.7	10.2 7.3	6.2 11.8	8.7	6.1 6	6.8 6.8	6.3 6.3	7.2	6.1	7.6	5.4
RR (bpm)	—	22.1 15.6	—	29 16	20	29 29	26 25.2	—	—	27	20.8	29.7
Peak (cm H_2O)	—	24.2 32.1	—	32 39	34	—	—	—	—		27	—
Plateau (cm H_2O)	25.7 31.7	22.3 26.8	30.6 24.9	25 33	28	24 27	24.9 30.2	23 29	26	23	23	27.9
PEEP (cm H_2O)	10.7 10.7	8.6 7.2	~8.2 ~9.5	9.4 8.6	8	8.9 14.7	10.1 15.6	9 15	9.3	10	8.5	16.4
Mortality (%)	46.6[b] 37.9[b]	47[c] 46[c]	50[c] 46[c]	31[c] 39.8[c]	52[c]	24.9[c] 27.5[c]	32.3[d] 28.4[d]	36.6[c] 30.3[c]	42.7[c]	32.8[d]	35.3[c]	55.3[d]

Abbreviations: PEEP, positive end-expiratory pressure; RCT, randomized controlled trial; RR, respiratory rate; V_t, tidal volume.
[a] Supine group only.
[b] Mortality: 14 days.
[c] Mortality: intensive care unit/hospital mortality.
[d] Mortality: 28 days.

with severe and moderate to severe ARDS).[33] Conversely, milder patients do not usually present major problems of VILI.

1. Respiratory mechanics. Before finally setting the ventilator, an accurate characterization of the patient should be available, including the measurements of mechanical characteristics, such as pulmonary and respiratory system elastance. These data are fundamental to estimate the mechanical power needed for ventilation.
2. Lung volumes. The measurement of the lung size (FRC) allows for an estimate of the total lung capacity and defines the limit of the area within which the mechanical ventilation is applied. Ideally, this measurement should be done by CT scan, which allows for the assessment of several other characteristics of the patient. Nonetheless, other techniques may also be used.
3. Consider that the risks of volutrauma are higher than the risks of atelectrauma. Therefore, it is not only unnecessary but even harmful to pursue a complete lung opening, which may occur at volume and pressure close to the unknown total lung capacity.
4. Whatever maneuver is performed, it should be associated with an assessment of the hemodynamic consequences.
5. Make the lung as homogeneous as possible to tolerate the mechanical ventilation. The best way to reach this goal is to pronate the patients.
6. Set the target of mechanical ventilation: a Pao_2 and $Paco_2$ of 60 mm Hg may be acceptable, compared with the "price" that has to be paid in pursuit of more normal values.

REFERENCES

1. Hayes DF, Lucas CE. Bilateral tube thoracostomy to preclude fatal tension pneumothorax in patients with acute respiratory insufficiency. Am Surg 1976; 42:330–1.
2. Kolobow T, Moretti MP, Fumagalli R, et al. Severe impairment in lung function induced by high peak airway pressure during mechanical ventilation. An experimental study. Am Rev Respir Dis 1987;135:312–5.
3. Gattinoni L, Carlesso E, Cadringher P, et al. Physical and biological triggers of ventilator-induced lung injury and its prevention. Eur Respir J Suppl 2003;47: 15s–25s.
4. Zapol WM, Snider MT, Hill JD, et al. Extracorporeal membrane oxygenation in severe acute respiratory failure. A randomized prospective study. JAMA 1979;242: 2193–6.
5. Dreyfuss D, Soler P, Basset G, et al. High inflation pressure pulmonary edema. Respective effects of high airway pressure, high tidal volume, and positive end-expiratory pressure. Am Rev Respir Dis 1988;137:1159–64.
6. Hickling KG, Henderson SJ, Jackson R. Low mortality associated with low volume pressure limited ventilation with permissive hypercapnia in severe adult respiratory distress syndrome. Intensive Care Med 1990;16:372–7.
7. Tremblay L, Valenza F, Ribeiro SP, et al. Injurious ventilatory strategies increase cytokines and c-fos m-RNA expression in an isolated rat lung model. J Clin Invest 1997;99:944–52.
8. Mead J, Takishima T, Leith D. Stress distribution in lungs: a model of pulmonary elasticity. J Appl Physiol 1970;28:596–608.
9. Lachmann B. Open up the lung and keep the lung open. Intensive Care Med 1992;18:319–21.

10. Amato MB, Barbas CS, Medeiros DM, et al. Effect of a protective-ventilation strategy on mortality in the acute respiratory distress syndrome. N Engl J Med 1998; 338:347–54.

11. Ranieri VM, Suter PM, Tortorella C, et al. Effect of mechanical ventilation on inflammatory mediators in patients with acute respiratory distress syndrome: a randomized controlled trial. JAMA 1999;282:54–61.

12. Gattinoni L, Marini JJ, Collino F, et al. The future of mechanical ventilation: lessons from the present and the past. Crit Care 2017;21:183.

13. Gattinoni L, Tonetti T, Cressoni M, et al. Ventilator-related causes of lung injury: the mechanical power. Intensive Care Med 2016;42:1567–75.

14. Cressoni M, Cadringher P, Chiurazzi C, et al. Lung inhomogeneity in patients with acute respiratory distress syndrome. Am J Respir Crit Care Med 2014;189: 149–58.

15. Schumann S, Goebel U, Haberstroh J, et al. Determination of respiratory system mechanics during inspiration and expiration by FLow-controlled EXpiration (FLEX): a pilot study in anesthetized pigs. Minerva Anestesiol 2014;80:19–28.

16. Caironi P, Langer T, Carlesso E, et al. Time to generate ventilator-induced lung injury among mammals with healthy lungs: a unifying hypothesis. Intensive Care Med 2011;37:1913–20.

17. Acute Respiratory Distress Syndrome Network, Brower RG, Matthay MA, Morris A, et al. Ventilation with lower tidal volumes as compared with traditional tidal volumes for acute lung injury and the acute respiratory distress syndrome. N Engl J Med 2000;342:1301–8.

18. Chiumello D, Cressoni M, Chierichetti M, et al. Nitrogen washout/washin, helium dilution and computed tomography in the assessment of end expiratory lung volume. Crit Care 2008;12:1–8.

19. Gattinoni L, Pesenti A. The concept of "baby lung". Intensive Care Med 2005;31: 776–84.

20. Meade MO, Cook DJ, Guyatt GH, et al, Lung open ventilation study Investigators. Ventilation strategy using low tidal volumes, recruitment maneuvers, and high positive end-expiratory pressure for acute lung injury and acute respiratory distress syndrome: a randomized controlled trial. JAMA 2008;299:637–45.

21. Mercat A, Richard JC, Vielle B, et al, Expiratory Pressure Study Group. Positive end-expiratory pressure setting in adults with acute lung injury and acute respiratory distress syndrome: a randomized controlled trial. JAMA 2008;299:646–55.

22. Brower RG, Lanken PN, MacIntyre N, et al. Higher versus lower positive end-expiratory pressures in patients with the acute respiratory distress syndrome. N Engl J Med 2004;351:327–36.

23. Writing Group for the Alveolar Recruitment for Acute Respiratory Distress Syndrome Trial Investigators, Cavalcanti AB, Suzumura EA, Laranjeira LN, et al. Effect of lung recruitment and titrated Positive End-Expiratory Pressure (PEEP) vs low peep on mortality in patients with acute respiratory distress syndrome: a randomized clinical trial. JAMA 2017;318:1335–45.

24. Esteban A, Anzueto A, Frutos F, et al, Mechanical Ventilation International Study Group. Characteristics and outcomes in adult patients receiving mechanical ventilation: a 28-day international study. JAMA 2002;287:345–55.

25. Villar J, Blanco J, Anon JM, et al. The ALIEN study: incidence and outcome of acute respiratory distress syndrome in the era of lung protective ventilation. Intensive Care Med 2011;37:1932–41.

26. Bellani G, Laffey JG, Pham T, et al. Epidemiology, patterns of care, and mortality for patients with acute respiratory distress syndrome in intensive care units in 50 countries. JAMA 2016;315:788–800.
27. Brochard L, Roudot-Thoraval F, Roupie E, et al. Tidal volume reduction for prevention of ventilator-induced lung injury in acute respiratory distress syndrome. The Multicenter Trail Group on Tidal Volume reduction in ARDS. Am J Respir Crit Care Med 1998;158:1831–8.
28. Stewart TE, Meade MO, Cook DJ, et al. Evaluation of a ventilation strategy to prevent barotrauma in patients at high risk for acute respiratory distress syndrome. Pressure- and volume-limited ventilation strategy group. N Engl J Med 1998;338:355–61.
29. Brower RG, Shanholtz CB, Fessler HE, et al. Prospective, randomized, controlled clinical trial comparing traditional versus reduced tidal volume ventilation in acute respiratory distress syndrome patients. Crit Care Med 1999;27:1492–8.
30. Guerin C, Reignier J, Richard JC, et al. Prone positioning in severe acute respiratory distress syndrome. N Engl J Med 2013;368:2159–68.
31. Young D, Lamb SE, Shah S, et al. High-frequency oscillation for acute respiratory distress syndrome. N Engl J Med 2013;368:806–13.
32. Ferguson ND, Cook DJ, Guyatt GH, et al, Canadian Critical Care Trials Group. High-frequency oscillation in early acute respiratory distress syndrome. N Engl J Med 2013;368:795–805.
33. Maiolo G, Collino F, Vasques F, et al. Reclassifying acute respiratory distress syndrome. Am J Respir Crit Care Med 2018. [Epub ahead of print].
34. Briel M, Meade M, Mercat A, et al. Higher vs lower positive end-expiratory pressure in patients with acute lung injury and acute respiratory distress syndrome: systematic review and meta-analysis. JAMA 2010;303:865–73.

Avoiding Respiratory and Peripheral Muscle Injury During Mechanical Ventilation

Diaphragm-Protective Ventilation and Early Mobilization

Annia Schreiber, MD[a], Michele Bertoni, MD[b],
Ewan C. Goligher, MD, PhD[c,d],*

KEYWORDS

- Limb muscle weakness • Respiratory muscle weakness • Ventilator dependence
- Intensive care unit • Mechanical ventilation

KEY POINTS

- Both limb muscle weakness and respiratory muscle weakness are exceedingly common in critically ill patients.
- Respiratory muscle weakness prolongs ventilator dependence, predisposing to nosocomial complications (including limb muscle weakness) and death.
- Limb muscle weakness persists for months after discharge from intensive care and results in poor long-term functional status and quality of life.
- Major mechanisms of muscle injury include critical illness polymyoneuropathy, sepsis, pharmacologic exposures, metabolic derangements, and excessive muscle loading and unloading.
- The diaphragm may become weak because of excessive unloading (leading to atrophy) or because of excessive loading (either concentric or eccentric) owing to excessive ventilator assistance.

---

[a] Respiratory Intensive Care Unit and Pulmonary Rehabilitation Unit, Istituti Clinici Scientifici Maugeri, Scientific Institute of Pavia, Via Salvatore Maugeri 10, Pavia 27100, Italy; [b] Department of Anesthesia, Critical Care and Emergency, Spedali Civili University Hospital, Piazzale Spedali Civili 1, Brescia 25123, Italy; [c] Interdepartmental Division of Critical Care Medicine, University of Toronto, Toronto, ON, Canada; [d] Division of Respirology, Department of Medicine, University Health Network, Toronto General Hospital, 585 University Avenue, Peter Munk Building, 11th Floor Room 192, Toronto, ON M5G 2N2, Canada
* Corresponding author. Mount Sinai Hospital, 600 University Avenue, Room 18-206, Toronto, ON M5G 1X5, Canada.
E-mail address: ewan.goligher@mail.utoronto.ca

Crit Care Clin 34 (2018) 357–381
https://doi.org/10.1016/j.ccc.2018.03.005
0749-0704/18/© 2018 Elsevier Inc. All rights reserved.

criticalcare.theclinics.com

INTRODUCTION

The introduction of positive-pressure ventilation in the mid-20th century led to the advent of the modern intensive care unit with all its previously unimagined possibilities for survival and recovery from severe life-threatening illness. Yet, as survival after critical illness has dramatically improved (general intensive care unit [ICU] mortality rates after acute respiratory failure are now estimated at 25%–30%[1]), attention has increasingly turned to the sequelae of critical illness in survivors. The impact of critical illness persists long after ICU discharge as survivors struggle with functional disability, cognitive impairment, and neuropsychiatric illness in the months and years after critical illness.

Muscle weakness affecting both the respiratory muscles and peripheral muscles of the axial skeleton is thought to be a key mediator of this protracted disability after critical illness. Limb muscle atrophy and dysfunction can persist for months after "recovery" from acute respiratory failure. Respiratory muscle weakness is a major risk factor for prolonged mechanical ventilation, a development that entails a grave risk of long-term morbidity and mortality. Muscle injury during critical illness is, therefore, a subject of vital importance.

This article provides an overview of the epidemiology, mechanisms of respiratory muscle and limb muscle weakness during critical illness, and impact of both forms of muscle weakness on clinical outcomes. We outline strategies to prevent and treat limb and respiratory muscle weakness in critically ill patients.

DEFINITION AND EPIDEMIOLOGY

Muscle weakness is defined as impairment in the force-generating capacity of muscle. Because the force generated by muscle tissue is correlated with the magnitude of the neural contractile stimulus, reliable muscle function assessment requires a standardized stimulus. Standardization is accomplished either by eliciting a maximal stimulus (eg, maximal contractile effort) or by applying a standardized nonvolitional stimulus (eg, twitch magnetic stimulation). Techniques for assessing muscle function in ICU patients are summarized in **Table 1**. These techniques are reviewed in detail elsewhere.[2,3] Clinicians should bear in mind that maximal volitional efforts may be difficult to obtain in critically ill patients owing to impaired consciousness, delirium, sedation, or central fatigue.

Respiratory Muscle Weakness

A substantial proportion of ICU patients—up to 80%—develop respiratory muscle weakness at some point during their ICU stay.[4,5] Diaphragm weakness is present in the majority of patients at ICU admission.[6,7] This early diaphragm weakness has been associated with markers of illness severity and is associated with an increased risk of death but not prolonged ventilation, suggesting that early diaphragm weakness represents a form of reversible organ failure related to the patient's critical illness.

In patients who are ready to commence the weaning phase of ventilation, the prevalence of diaphragm weakness varies between 63% and 80%.[8–10] Estimates of the prevalence of diaphragm weakness are somewhat lower when diaphragm ultrasound examination is used to assess diaphragm function, ranging between 29% in patients submitted to the first spontaneous breathing trial[11] and 36% in prolonged weaning patients.[12,13]

These rather dramatic prevalence estimates are corroborated by histologic studies of diaphragm biopsies obtained from brain dead organ donors and mechanically

| Table 1 ||||
| Techniques for evaluating limb and respiratory muscle strength in the clinical setting ||||

Technique	Pros	Cons	Cutoff for Weakness
Respiratory muscles			
Ultrasound imaging			
Diaphragm excursion	Highly reproducible Feasible at the bedside Noninvasive	Requires patient volitional effort Difficult to visualize in some patients (bowel gas) Confounded by the effects of mechanical ventilation on lung inflation (needs to be measured on CPAP)	<1 cm[11]
Diaphragm maximal thickening fraction	Highly feasible at the bedside Noninvasive Shown to predict the risk of weaning failure[114]	Requires patient volitional effort Reproducibility uncertain	<20%[115]
Pressures			
Maximal inspiratory pressure	Simple maneuver Feasible at the bedside	Requires full cooperation and coordination (may be difficult in critically ill patients) Results often underestimated	Age- and sex-specific values[116]
Sniff inspiratory pressure	Simple maneuver Feasible at the bedside Provides highly reproducible results	Can be difficult in ventilated patients (uncertain)	Age and sex-specific values[117]
Transdiaphragmatic pressure	Avoids confounding from abdominal muscle activity	Requires insertion of esophageal and gastric balloon catheters	Pdi,max <60 cm H_2O[118]
Gilbert index ($\Delta Pga/\Delta Pdi$)	Simple maneuver	Requires insertion of esophageal and gastric balloon catheters Incorrect placement of the gastric balloon in the lower esophagus and recruitment of abdominal muscles mimic severe weakness	<0[118]

(continued on next page)

Table 1
(continued)

Technique	Pros	Cons	Cutoff for Weakness
Magnetic phrenic nerve stimulation	Provides a standardized measure independent of the patient's volitional effort Feasible in sedated patients	Requires magnetic stimulation (expensive) Requires considerable operator expertise Serial stimulation may not be well-tolerated	Pdi,tw < −10 cm H_2O[118] Paw,tw < −11 cm H_2O[119]
Neuromuscular coupling	May be independent of volitional effort (uncertain) Assess the mechanical performance of the muscle Shown to be a predictor of extubation success/failure when measured during SBT[120]	Requires insertion of nasogastric catheter and specialized equipment Reproducibility uncertain	
Limb muscles			
MRC score	Simple, intuitive and good interobserver reliability Feasible at the bedside Noninvasive	Requires patient cooperation May be compromised by pain, sedation, delirium, altered mental status It does not evaluate distal extremity function (eg, intrinsic hand muscles, the first affected in neuropathies)	MRC score < 48 (or mean score of <4 per muscle group)[5]
Hand dynamometry	Highly feasible at the bedside Noninvasive	Requires voluntary muscle contraction May be compromised by pain, sedation, delirium, altered mental status	<11 kg-force for men <7 kg-force for women[121]
Ultrasound imaging (quantitative: muscle mass; qualitative: myofiber necrosis)	Feasible and reliable Noninvasive	Probably underestimates the muscle loss	No single threshold diagnostic of weakness (10% threshold frequently used)[122]

(continued on next page)

Technique	Pros	Cons	Cutoff for Weakness
Table 1 *(continued)*			
Magnetic femoral nerve stimulation	Good reproducibility[123] Well-tolerated	Difficult to perform in ventilated patients Recent studies have shown a knee support could increase feasibility in critically ill patients	Clinically significant values have to be defined in critically ill patients
Conventional nerve conduction studies and electromyography	Provide specific anatomic diagnosis of etiology of weakness Minimally invasive	Technically challenging, requires specialized personal	See diagnostic criteria for critical illness polyneuropathy and myopathy[124]
Simplified electrophysiologic testing: peroneal nerve test	Highly feasible at the bedside Validated in a single study Nonvolitional Minimally invasive Can be used as a screening tool	Cannot distinguish between CIP, CIM, or both	Maximum peak-to-peak CMAP amplitude < 5 mV suggests neuropathy[125]

Abbreviations: CIM, critical illness myopathy; CIP, critical illness polyneuropathy; CMAP, compound muscle action potential; CPAP, continuous positive airway pressure; MRC, Medical Research Council; Paw,tw, twitch airway pressure; Pdi,max, maximal transdiaphragmatic pressure; Pdi,tw, twitch transdiaphragmatic pressure; SBT, spontaneous breathing trial.

ventilated patients. Structural abnormalities—atrophy, inflammation, and sarcomeric disarray—are nearly universal in these tissue samples.[14–16]

Importantly, the expiratory muscles—crucial for cough strength and augmenting diaphragm function[17]—are also affected. One study found that maximal expiratory pressure tended to be significantly reduced (median of 30 cm H_2O) in patients after 1 week of ventilation.[18]

Limb Muscle Weakness

Between 25% and 55% of mechanically ventilated patients develop severe limb muscle weakness.[3,19,20] The prevalence and severity of limb muscle weakness increases significantly with the duration of ventilation. The majority of patients who require prolonged ventilation (>7 days) exhibit marked limb muscle weakness,[18] and electrophysiologic studies have demonstrated diffuse neuromuscular abnormalities in more than 50% of ICU patients after 5 to 7 days of mechanical ventilation.[21,22]

Because the usual tool for assessing limb muscle function (the Medical Research Council scale) requires volitional participation, there is a relative paucity of data on limb muscle strength during the early course of the ICU stay. Quadriceps thickness progressively decreases by 10% to 20% over the first 7 to 10 days of mechanical ventilation in association with significant decreases in the muscle fiber cross-sectional area.[23] The rate of decrease in thickness is considerably greater in patients with multiorgan failure (vs single organ failure), suggesting that, as with early respiratory muscle weakness, critical illness per se is a primary driver of limb muscle weakness.

Respiratory Muscle Weakness and Limb Muscle Weakness: Not the Same Disease

Although it is often assumed that limb and respiratory muscle weakness constitute the same disease process, several considerations suggest that they should be regarded as independent phenomena.

First, the time course of structural change in the muscle differs markedly between the 2 groups. Whereas quadriceps muscle thickness decreased by about 10% after 1 week of ventilation, diaphragm atrophy is considerably more rapid,[24,25] with 50% of patients losing a median of 20% of diaphragm thickness by day 3 or 4 of mechanical ventilation. Diaphragm atrophy occurs earlier and is much more profound than limb muscle atrophy.

Second, at the commencement of the weaning phase, respiratory muscle weakness is only very weakly correlated with peripheral muscle weakness. Dres and colleagues[3] demonstrated that diaphragm weakness was much more common than peripheral muscle weakness at that time point; only 21% of patients exhibited both diaphragm weakness and peripheral muscle weakness. De Jonghe and colleagues[18] demonstrated a slightly stronger correlation later in the course of critical illness. This relative lack of correlation and the marked difference in prevalence suggest that different mechanisms acting at different points in time give rise to respiratory and peripheral muscle weakness.

CLINICAL SIGNIFICANCE: IMPACT ON OUTCOMES

Muscle weakness is strongly linked to poor short-term and long-term clinical outcomes for mechanically ventilated patients, but these epidemiologic associations must be interpreted with caution because muscle weakness is also strongly linked to severity of illness and the risk of unmeasured confounding is, therefore, not insignificant.

Respiratory Muscle Weakness

The association between respiratory muscle weakness and clinical outcome varies over the time course of critical illness. The presence of diaphragm weakness at the time of admission predicts an increased risk of mortality, but is not related to the duration of ventilation.[7] Presumably, this early weakness represents a reversible form of organ failure related to the primary critical illness that recovers as the illness resolves.

In contrast, respiratory muscle weakness at the commencement of weaning is strongly associated with the duration of ventilation and the risk of difficult or prolonged weaning from mechanical ventilation.[8,11,26] The presence of respiratory muscle weakness at ICU discharge predicts a significantly higher risk of death or readmission to the ICU or hospital.[27,28]

Structural changes in the diaphragm associated with mechanical ventilation also predict poor clinical outcomes.[29] The development of diaphragm atrophy during ventilation is associated OR in association with prolonged duration of ventilation, prolonged ICU admission, and a markedly higher risk of complications of acute respiratory failure, including reintubation and tracheostomy.

Peripheral Muscle Weakness

Several studies have found that the development of limb muscle weakness is associated with prolonged mechanical ventilation, increased health care costs, and an increased risk of death after hospital discharge.[18–20] Peripheral muscle weakness present at ICU discharge often persists for months afterward[30,31] and this persistent weakness is in turn associated with long-term physical disability.[30,32]

Because most of these studies diagnosed ICU-acquired weakness later in the course of critical illness at or near ICU discharge, it is uncertain whether limb muscle weakness leads to prolonged ventilation, or vice versa. Recently, Dres and colleagues[8] demonstrated that limb muscle weakness present at the first spontaneous breathing trial was not associated with prolonged ventilation, in contrast with respiratory muscle weakness (**Fig. 1**). This finding suggests that respiratory muscle weakness drives prolonged mechanical ventilation, which in turn increases the risk of developing persistent limb muscle weakness and associated long-term disability (**Fig. 2**). Thus, preventing respiratory muscle weakness and accelerating liberation from mechanical ventilation might, in fact, prevent limb muscle weakness and attendant morbidity.

MECHANISMS OF MUSCLE INJURY AND WEAKNESS DURING CRITICAL ILLNESS

A wide range of factors contribute to muscle injury and weakness in the context of critical illness. Herein we provide a summary of these factors, focusing especially on those mechanisms offering potential targets for intervention. These mechanisms are summarized in **Fig. 3**.

Critical Illness Polymyoneuropathy

First described in the 1980s by Bolton and colleagues,[33] critical illness polymyoneuropathy is now widely recognized as an important cause of ICU-acquired muscle weakness affecting both the limb and respiratory muscles.[34] The neuropathy component is characterized by axonal degeneration without demyelination. The myopathy is

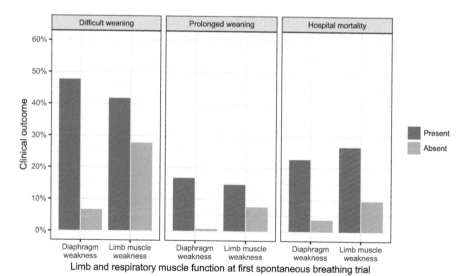

Fig. 1. Diaphragm weakness predicts adverse clinical outcomes much more strongly than limb muscle weakness at the time of the first spontaneous breathing trial. The risk of difficult weaning, prolonged weaning, and death in hospital were significantly higher in patients with diaphragm weakness (based on twitch magnetic phrenic stimulation) compared with those in patients without diaphragm weakness. The differences in risk were much smaller between patients with and without limb muscle weakness (based on Medical Research Council score). (*Data from* Dres M, Dube BP, Mayaux J, et al. Coexistence and impact of limb muscle and diaphragm weakness at time of liberation from mechanical ventilation in medical intensive care unit patients. Am J Respir Crit Care Med 2017;195(1):57–66.)

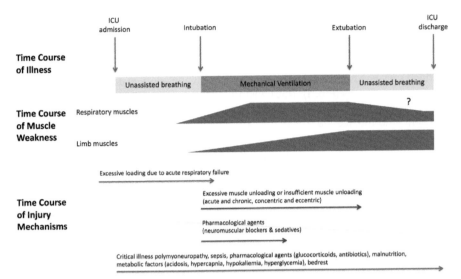

Fig. 2. Time course of limb and respiratory muscle weakness during mechanical ventilation. Respiratory muscle weakness develops more rapidly than limb muscle weakness. Its influence on outcome is greater at an early stage (see **Fig. 1**). The development of respiratory muscle weakness and prolonged ventilator-dependence permit greater time for the development of limb muscle weakness and associated poor long-term outcomes. Mechanisms of injury at various time points are shown. ICU, intensive care unit.

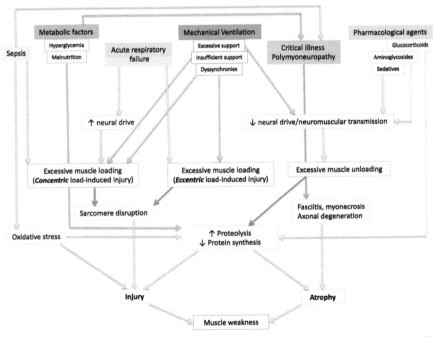

Fig. 3. Mechanisms of injury to the limb and respiratory muscles during mechanical ventilation. See text for details.

characterized by atrophy, fasciitis, and myonecrosis. Patients may exhibit either or both neuropathy and myopathy, and those with multiorgan failure are especially likely to be affected.[23] Both the nerve and muscle injuries likely represent the downstream effects of many mechanisms including excessive unloading, sepsis and systemic inflammation, microvascular ischemia, and metabolic derangements (particularly hyperglycemia).[35] We, therefore, explore each of these specific mechanisms in more detail.

Excessive Muscle Unloading

The deleterious effects of prolonged immobility and bedrest on muscle structure and function have long been recognized.[36] In critically ill patients, the muscles are often completely unloaded for a period of time owing to the effects of sedation, paralysis, and mechanical ventilatory support. Both limb muscle atrophy and diaphragm atrophy are well-described complications of this unloading. It is important to recognize that muscle atrophy is not the consequence of inactivity per se, but rather results from a decrease in tension generated within the myofibril (ie, the load on the muscle).[37]

Muscle unloading leads to atrophy by upregulation in proteolytic systems and downregulation of protein synthetic systems, giving rise to atrophy in both the limb and respiratory muscles.[38] Interestingly, the means by which mechanical forces on the myofibril are transduced to biological signals remains uncertain; some evidence suggests that titin—a major structural protein in the myofibril—might act as a mechanosensor.[39] Observations in animal models and brain-dead organ donors suggested that mitochondrial dysfunction in the diaphragm might trigger oxidative stress and proteolysis,[40] although a recent study found no evidence of mitochondrial dysfunction in atrophic diaphragm tissue obtained from live patients early during the course of mechanical ventilation.[15]

Diaphragm atrophy

If the pressure and flow delivered by the mechanical ventilator unload the diaphragm excessively, diaphragm atrophy and weakness rapidly develop.[16,25,41] Experimental studies in a range of animal models have demonstrated that diaphragm unloading under controlled mechanical ventilation and/or pressure support (at high levels of assist) rapidly leads to diaphragm atrophy, myofibril injury, and weakness.[42–46]

Diaphragm disuse atrophy has been extensively documented in the clinical setting. Histologic specimens of the diaphragm obtained from brain-dead organ donors[16,40,41,47] and live mechanically ventilated patients[14,48] consistently exhibit a pattern of atrophy and injury similar to that of animal models. Imaging studies using ultrasound imaging and computed tomography scanning have demonstrated progressive atrophy over time.[10,24,25,49] Diaphragm thickness may decrease by as much as 30% to 40% over 3 days in some patients.[50] The rate of atrophy is inversely proportional to the level of diaphragm loading (inspiratory effort) assessed by diaphragm ultrasound imaging.[50] These morphologic changes are clinically significant: decreases in diaphragm thickness were associated with impaired diaphragm function and a higher risk of prolonged mechanical ventilation, reintubation, and tracheostomy.[29]

Limb muscle atrophy

The limb muscles are often completely unloaded for prolonged periods of time in critically ill patients owing to prolonged immobilization; yet, limb muscle atrophy develops more slowly than diaphragm atrophy.[42,44] Using serial ultrasound imaging,

Puthucheary and colleagues[51] found that rectus femoris cross-sectional area decreased by approximately 10% over the first week of mechanical ventilation. Atrophy proceeded more rapidly in patients with a greater number of failing organs. The degree of atrophy and the balance of protein synthesis and breakdown was correlated to the severity of systemic inflammation; the level of mobility was not measured, but the authors speculated that differences in mobility level were unlikely to account for the observed variation in rates of atrophy. In general, the degree of muscle wasting in critically ill patients exceeds that expected from complete muscle unloading, suggesting the importance of additional factors driving net protein loss.

In a cohort study of survivors of critical illness, quadriceps muscle atrophy was present in all patients 7 days after ICU discharge.[30] The regrowth of muscle over the ensuing months varied considerably between patients, but most patients still had atrophy 6 months after ICU discharge. Interestingly, even those patients who regained muscle bulk remained quite weak, although the mechanism of this weakness was unclear.

Excessive Muscle Loading

Although the harms of muscle disuse are now widely recognized, the deleterious effects of excessive muscle loading are less well-appreciated. In fact, evidence is beginning to mount that excess loading may give rise to clinically significant respiratory muscle injury. Two forms of excess loading may be distinguished: concentric and eccentric.

Concentric load-induced injury

Concentric load-induced injury results when muscular contraction and shortening generates an injuriously high level of tension within the muscle. Sustained high inspiratory resistive loading leads to marked diaphragm injury, inflammation, weakness.[52] The injured diaphragm exhibits sarcomeric disruption and myofibrillar susceptibility to calpain-mediated degradation.[53]

Although the threshold for load-induced diaphragm injury in humans is usually relatively high,[54] critically ill patients may be much more susceptible to load-induced injury because systemic inflammation renders the sarcolemma fragile and more vulnerable to injury from mechanical stress.[55] Indeed, in an animal model of sepsis, diaphragm inactivity during mechanical ventilation prevented muscle membrane injury and diaphragm weakness compared with spontaneous breathing.[56]

Both acute and chronic resistive overloading lead to diaphragm injury in humans.[57] Diaphragm biopsy specimens in mechanically ventilated patients exhibit significant inflammatory infiltration and sarcomeric disarray, similar to that seen in models of load-induced injury.[15,47] Given that high respiratory effort levels are frequently observed in mechanically ventilated patients owing to high respiratory drive, inadequate ventilator support, and patient–ventilator dyssynchrony, critically ill patients are likely at risk of load-induced diaphragm injury.

Concerns over excessive diaphragm loading are circumstantially supported by the recent observation that some ventilated patients develop a rapid increase in diaphragm thickness during the early course of ventilation in association with relatively high levels of inspiratory effort.[29] Patients who developed this increase in thickness tended to have impaired diaphragm function and were more likely to require prolonged mechanical ventilation, supporting the possibility that such increases in diaphragm thickness reflected load-induced muscle injury. Biceps cross-sectional area increased acutely after load-induced injury[58]; it is unknown whether this is also the case for the diaphragm.

Eccentric load-induced injury

Eccentric contractions during muscular lengthening are considerably more injurious than concentric contractions during muscular shortening.[59] Eccentric contractions increase the tension applied to the muscle for a given level of pressure generation[60] and eccentric diaphragm loading was shown to cause significant acute diaphragm injury in an experimental model.[61]

Normal subjects generally exhibit low levels of eccentric contraction during resting tidal ventilation.[62] More vigorous eccentric contractions may occur under several conditions related to critical illness. First, when respiratory mechanical loads are increased, diaphragm contractile activity during expiration ("expiratory braking") mitigates against the worsening of atelectasis.[63,64] Second, the diaphragm may contract eccentrically during certain forms of patient–ventilator dyssynchrony that result in patient inspiratory effort during the expiratory phase when lung volume is decreasing and the diaphragm is lengthening. Such forms of dyssynchrony include ineffective efforts, where the patient is unable to trigger the ventilator,[65] and reverse triggering,[66] where neural inspiration results from passive mechanical inflation and often extends into mechanical expiration.

Sepsis

Infection is a major risk factor for the development of marked diaphragm weakness in mechanically ventilated patients.[7,67] Diaphragm strength was decreased by approximately 50% in patients with sepsis compared with patients without sepsis.[7] Muscle weakness associated with sepsis is mediated by proinflammatory cytokines, oxidative stress, and the activation of proteolytic pathways.[68] Sepsis also impairs both oxygen delivery and use at the cellular level, leading to deranged metabolism and contractile dysfunction.[3] As discussed, sepsis increases muscle membrane fragility, heightening sensitivity to the injurious effects of loading. In this respect, the bedrest and temporary immobilization associated with sepsis may constitute an adaptive (rather than a maladaptive) response to systemic infection.

Pharmacologic Agents

Many medications used to treat critically ill patients have myopathic effects.[69] Sedatives can exert both direct injurious effects and indirect effects by promoting rest and disuse atrophy. Propofol causes a dose-related decrease in diaphragm contractility.[70] Neuromuscular blockade may contribute to disuse and consequent atrophy as well. Of note, aminosteroidal paralytic agents (eg, rocuronium) have greater myopathic effects than benzylisoquinoline agents (eg, cisatracurium), possibly as a consequence of its glucocorticoid-like effects on intracellular calcium homeostasis and proteolysis.[71] This class effect may account for the absence of any difference in limb muscle weakness in the largest randomized trial of a neuromuscular blocking agent (cisatracurium) in mechanically ventilated patients with acute respiratory distress syndrome.[72]

Glucocorticoid agents, commonly used in the ICU, are a well-known cause of skeletal muscle myopathy involving both respiratory and peripheral muscles. Glucocorticoids inhibit protein synthesis and activate proteolysis.[73] However, the effects of glucocorticoids are complex and likely depend to some extent on the specific agent, the dose, and the patient's condition. Maes and colleagues[74] reported that, counterintuitively, high-dose methylprednisolone administered during controlled ventilation prevented calpain activation and inhibited calpase-3, thereby protecting against the development of ventilator-induced diaphragm dysfunction. In contrast, low-dose methylprednisolone was even more deleterious than controlled mechanical ventilation alone.

Certain antibiotic agents may exacerbate muscle weakness. Aminoglycosides interfere with neuromuscular transmission.[69]

Metabolic Factors

A variety of metabolic derangements associated with critical illness can exacerbate muscle weakness. Respiratory acidosis, hypercapnia, and hypokalemia contribute to reversible diaphragm weakness, whereas metabolic acidosis seems to have no effect.[75] At the same time, however, hypercapnia may protect against the development of ventilator-induced diaphragmatic dysfunction.[76,77] Hyperglycemia is an important modifiable risk factor for muscle injury.[78] Chronic malnutrition predisposes to ICU-acquired weakness owing to a lack of muscle protein reserves at baseline.[79]

PREVENTION AND TREATMENT

Respiratory and limb muscle weakness is an important clinical problem. Having summarized the key mechanisms of muscle injury and weakness, we are better positioned to understand how such efforts should be undertaken. Strategies for prevention and treatment are summarized in **Table 2**.

General Supportive Care

Perhaps the most effective strategy to avoid the development of limb and respiratory muscle weakness is to minimize the duration of critical illness by timely diagnosis, resuscitation, and therapy of the underlying cause of critical illness. Sepsis in particular requires rapid assessment and appropriate therapy. Metabolic derangements, including electrolyte abnormalities, should be corrected. Neuromuscular blocking agents and corticosteroids should be administered judiciously and discontinued as soon as it is safe and clinically prudent to do so. Sedation should be managed according to established evidence-based strategies with the goal of minimizing chemical immobilization.[80] If continuous sedative infusions are necessary, short-acting titratable agents such as propofol are preferable over benzodiazepines (long context-sensitive half-life) to minimize immobility.[80] Pain and dyspnea should be aggressively controlled to facilitate mobilization. Close attention should be paid to glycemic control. Weaning practices should be standardized and the need for ongoing mechanical ventilation should be reevaluated on a daily basis.

Early Mobilization

Given that excessive muscle unloading is a key mechanism of muscle injury and weakness, great emphasis has been placed on mobilizing the patient as early as possible to mitigate against this mechanism of injury. Patients on mechanical ventilation (and even those on extracorporeal life support) can be safely mobilized out of bed.[81,82] The benefits of passive range-of-motion exercise should not be underestimated—generating tension within the muscle in the absence of active contraction significantly mitigates muscle atrophy.[83]

Despite a promising rationale, the impact of early mobilization on clinical outcomes seems to be limited—several randomized trials have yielded different results. Schweickert and colleagues[84] reported that early physical and occupational therapy during respiratory failure resulted in a higher rate of functional independence at hospital discharge. Unfortunately, this result has not translated into improvements in duration of ventilation, duration of hospitalization, long-term functional status, or quality of life as shown in several subsequent trials.[85–87] Differences in the outcomes of these various trials may relate to the timing, duration, and intensity of physical therapy, as

Table 2
Strategies for preventing and treating limb and respiratory muscle weakness

Strategy	Level of Evidence	Clinical Recommendations
Respiratory muscles		
Diaphragm-protective mechanical ventilation	Low (experimental and clinical data provide supportive rationale)	Optimizing synchrony and inspiratory load might prevent diaphragm injury Not yet for routine practice[29]
Inspiratory muscle training	Moderate (clinical data)	Both strength and endurance training techniques might result in a significant improvement in muscle strength, and shorten the duration of weaning and length of ICU stay[94] Consider using in selected patients at high risk of diaphragm weakness Can substantially improve outcomes after cardiac surgery when initiated preoperatively[126]
Pharmacologic agents Theophylline Levosimendan	Low (experimental and clinical data)	Enhance diaphragm contractility Not yet for routine practice
Limb muscles		
Early mobilization and rehabilitation	High (clinical data)	Improves muscle strength and mobility at time of discharge from hospital; no clear impact on long-term functional status or quality of life[89]
Respiratory and limb muscles		
Sedation limitation	Moderate (clinical data)	Maintaining light levels of sedation in adult ICU patients is associated with improved outcomes Shorter duration of mechanical ventilation and a shorter ICU duration of stay[80]
Glycemic control	Moderate (experimental and clinical data)	Glycemic control prevents muscle weakness[127]
Pharmacologic agents Antioxidants (N-acetylcysteina)	Low (experimental data)	Not in routine practice

Abbreviation: ICU, intensive care unit.

well as to control group management, because the field rapidly evolved to emphasize sedation minimization and early mobilization. Target population may be important: an early mobilization strategy specifically tested in surgical ICU patients accelerated ICU discharge and improved mobility at hospital discharge.[88]

A systematic review of the literature concluded that early mobilization improves limb muscle strength and mobility at hospital discharge, but these benefits did not translate into significant improvements in functional status, quality of life, or time to recovery.[89]

Clearly, more work is required to understand the role of unloading in the development of muscle weakness; it is possible that other mechanisms affecting the balance of protein synthesis and loss predominate over unloading. Furthermore, the interaction between the inflammatory state—which modulates the risk of load-induced injury—and the effect of mobilization needs careful study. It may not be safe to exercise inflamed muscle.

On the whole, these data suggest that clinicians should continue to minimize sedative use and bedrest, and to safely and carefully reload the limb muscles to improve muscle strength, recognizing the limited impact this may have on long-term quality of life. Excessive or unnecessary bedrest remains an important danger.

Diaphragm-Protective Mechanical Ventilation

The concept of diaphragm-protective ventilation arises from the notion that diaphragm injury results from either excessive unloading or excessive loading. As discussed, there is convincing evidence from multiple studies that the rate of change in diaphragm thickness is directly related to the degree of diaphragm loading or unloading and the manner in which the ventilator is set. This finding suggests that optimizing the load on the diaphragm (not too little and not too much) might prevent diaphragm injury and accelerate liberation from mechanical ventilation. The concept of diaphragm-protective ventilation is summarized in **Fig. 4**.

Diaphragm-protective ventilation has been studied in a porcine animal model. Jung and colleagues[90] applied controlled ventilation or adaptive support ventilation (a partially assisted mode of ventilation used a closed loop algorithm titrating ventilator support to optimize work of breathing based on the Otis equation) in porcine model of ventilator-induced diaphragmatic dysfunction. Animals in the adaptive support group did not develop diaphragm atrophy or weakness. This model has some limitations: unlike patients in the clinical setting, the animals had normal respiratory mechanics and respiratory drive was not elevated. But this study demonstrated that, in principle, mechanical ventilation can be adjusted to prevent diaphragm injury.

Diaphragm-protective ventilation has not yet been studied in humans and certain key questions remain. First, the optimal level of diaphragm loading is uncertain. Several competing factors may modify the safety of patient inspiratory effort, including

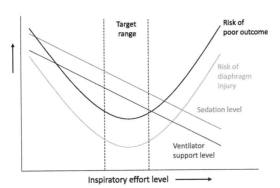

Fig. 4. Conceptual model of diaphragm-protective ventilation. Under this model, both insufficient and excessive inspiratory effort lead to deleterious structural and functional changes in the diaphragm, perpetuating ventilator-dependence and worsening clinical outcomes. Inspiratory effort is inversely related to the level of ventilator support and sedation. Targeting an intermediate level of inspiratory effort using carefully titrated levels of sedation and ventilator support can achieve a finely tuned optimal state that may prevent diaphragm injury and accelerate liberation from ventilation. (*Data from* Goligher EC, Dres M, Fan E, et al. Mechanical ventilation–induced diaphragm atrophy strongly impacts clinical outcomes. Am J Respir Crit Care Med 2018;197(2):204–13.)

hemodynamic shock states (where oxygen delivery may be compromised) and acute respiratory distress syndrome (where spontaneous respiratory effort may further propagate lung injury). Second, it is unclear whether respiratory drive and effort can be manipulated by ventilator support and sedation to achieve the target level of loading. Respiratory effort is often independent of chemoreceptive control in severely ill patients[91] and heavy sedation and paralysis may be necessary to control respiratory effort. Respiratory drive may be a "brittle" all or nothing phenomenon in these cases. One proposed solution is to implement partial neuromuscular blockade,[92] but this strategy has yet to be incorporated into a clinical protocol. Extracorporeal CO_2 removal may also provide a means of manipulating respiratory drive.[93]

Recent work suggests that the optimal diaphragm load may be similar to that of healthy subjects breathing at rest.[29] This level of respiratory effort was associated with relatively minimal changes in diaphragm thickness over time and predicted the shortest duration of ventilation compared with lower or high levels of effort. The feasibility and impact of titrating ventilator support (and sedation) to achieve this level of effort remain to be studied. To be effective, diaphragm-protective ventilation strategies must likely be implemented within 24 to 48 hours of initiating mechanical ventilation because much of the diaphragm atrophy and injury occur within 2 to 3 days of intubation.

Because patient–ventilator dyssynchrony may contribute to injurious diaphragm loading, monitoring and maintaining synchrony will be an essential feature of any diaphragm-protective ventilation strategy. The role of positive end-expiratory pressure also needs to be studied: a higher positive end-expiratory pressure may reduce diaphragm eccentric contractile activity associated with expiratory braking.

To achieve both synchrony and optimal respiratory effort, direct monitoring of the respiratory muscles is required. A range of monitoring strategies are available, including diaphragm electrical activity, diaphragm ultrasound, airway occlusion pressure measurement, and the classical technique of esophageal manometry. To implement diaphragm-protective ventilation, clinicians should familiarize themselves with 1 or more of these techniques.

In summary, diaphragm-protective ventilation is an extremely promising concept. Strategies to implement this approach in the clinical setting remain to be worked out. Because the optimal degree of diaphragm loading is likely to vary over time, further clinical investigation is necessary to characterize the relevant effects of diaphragm loading on the respiratory and cardiovascular systems before larger trials of diaphragm-protective ventilation are conducted.

Respiratory Muscle Rehabilitation and Inspiratory Muscle Training

Physical rehabilitation strategies for the limb muscles have received a great deal of attention. Yet, despite the high prevalence and serious clinical impact of respiratory muscle weakness, respiratory muscle rehabilitation has been largely neglected. Nevertheless, a number of studies have evaluated strategies for strengthening the respiratory muscles during mechanical ventilation.

Inspiratory muscle training involves applying a transiently increased inspiratory load to the respiratory muscles using flow resistance or threshold loading. Similar to autopositive end-expiratory pressure, externally applied threshold loading requires the patient to generate sufficient inspiratory pressure to reach a set threshold before inspiratory flow commences. It is, therefore, independent of inspiratory flow and patient inspiratory effort, an advantage that makes it easier to titrate reliably. Threshold loading devices are available; a threshold load can also be applied by manipulating the pressure trigger threshold on the ventilator.

The impact of inspiratory muscle training on clinical outcomes in mechanically ventilated patients was evaluated in a recent systematic review.[94] Training interventions included isocapnic/normocapnic hyperpnea, inspiratory resistive training, threshold load training, or the adjustment of ventilator pressure trigger sensitivity. In that review, inspiratory muscle training resulted in a significant improvement in maximum inspiratory pressure and in the likelihood of weaning and a reduction in the duration of stay. Training was well-tolerated, safe (no significant adverse events or complications), and feasible.

Loading techniques have been implemented at varying loads, frequencies, and durations. The optimal training strategy (intensity, duration, frequency) requires further study. Possibly, as mentioned, an optimal training protocol should include both intermediate loads and shortening velocities that allow patients to elicit improvements in both strength and endurance.[95] Caution is warranted to avoid load-induced muscle injury. The possibility of incorporating expiratory muscle training to enhance cough strength and augment ventilation also requires further investigation.

Neuromuscular Electrical Stimulation

Neuromuscular electrical stimulation (NMES) provides a means of loading muscle apart from patient volitional effort.

Neuromuscular electrical stimulation for respiratory muscle weakness
Given the challenges of controlling respiratory drive (particularly to maintain lung-protective ventilation), deep sedation is sometimes necessary. In this setting, external stimulation by diaphragmatic pacing offers an alternative means of avoiding excessive diaphragm unloading.

A preliminary case report of a patient with high spinal cord injury demonstrated that brief periods of unilateral electrical phrenic nerve stimulation (30 min/d) were enough to prevent diaphragm atrophy on the side of stimulation. Conversely, atrophy occurred on the side that failed to be stimulated owing to the removal of a phrenic nerve pacemaker.[96]

Phrenic nerve stimulation to pace the diaphragm during cardiovascular surgery was shown to prevent mitochondrial dysfunction[97] and maintain diaphragm contractility.[98] Phrenic nerve pacing delivered via a novel central venous catheter mitigated diaphragm atrophy during mechanical ventilation in a porcine experimental model[99] and this technique seems to be feasible in humans.[100]

Neuromuscular electrical stimulation for limb muscle weakness
NMES prevents quadriceps atrophy during prolonged immobilization in outpatients.[101] The role of NMES to prevent limb muscle weakness in the ICU remains the subject of active investigation. Studies reported to date suggest that NMES can maintain muscle physiology and strength, and prevent atrophy.[102] The functional impact of NMES remains uncertain, as does the optimal strategy for applying stimulation (dose, timing, etc). Patients with sepsis, edema, or shock are less likely to exhibit a significant muscular contraction in response to NMES.[103]

Nutrition

Hermans and coworkers[104] assessed the impact of 2 different nutritional strategies on muscle structure and function. Patients were randomized to receive early versus late parenteral nutrition (<2 days and <8 days after ICU admission). Surprisingly, the macronutrient deficiency in the first week experienced with the late regimen was not associated with significant fiber atrophy and, in contrast, seemed to improve muscle contractility. The increased autophagy observed in the late group probably plays an important beneficial role in protein turnover.

Pharmacologic Agents

To date, there are no drugs with established and accepted benefit for preventing or treating muscle weakness in mechanically ventilated patients. However, a number of drugs have a promising rationale for benefit, although few have been tested in humans.

In animal models, oxidative stress is a key mediator of ventilator-induced diaphragm dysfunction. Antioxidant agents prevent the development of diaphragm weakness during ventilation in these models[105,106] and in healthy subjects with diaphragm fatigue induced by inspiratory resistive loading.[107] High-dose (but not low-dose) corticosteroids administered during controlled ventilation reduced oxidative stress and prevented diaphragm atrophy in an animal model.[74]

Although neuromuscular blockade may cause diaphragm atrophy by unloading the respiratory muscles, the benefit of unloading may outweigh the harm if the patient is particularly at risk for load-induced injury. Consequently, neuromuscular blockade might actually limit respiratory muscle injury in patients with a very high respiratory drive, systemic inflammation predisposing to load-induced injury, and/or frequent patient–ventilator dyssynchronies resulting in eccentric contractions. This potential benefit has yet to be demonstrated.

Anabolic hormones can be used to enhance muscle protein content. Growth hormone has direct anabolic effects on skeletal muscle, but when high doses were administered to critically ill patients, growth hormone significantly increased the rates of multiorgan failure and mortality.[108] Testosterone, together with high caloric feeding, significantly improved inspiratory muscle strength in patients with stable chronic obstructive pulmonary disease,[109] but no data are available in ventilated ICU patients—many of whom have very low testosterone levels.[110]

Positive inotropes can enhance diaphragm contractility. Theophylline enhances diaphragm contractility in patients with diaphragm weakness,[111] but its narrow therapeutic range limits its utility. The calcium sensitizer levosimendan was able to improve neuromechanical efficiency and diaphragm contractile function in healthy subjects[112] and showed promising effects in patients with chronic obstructive pulmonary disease.[113] There are no trials to date in mechanically ventilated patients.

SUMMARY

Respiratory and limb muscle weakness is exceedingly common in mechanically ventilated patients and profoundly affects important clinical outcomes, including duration of mechanical ventilation, durations of stay in the ICU and hospital, risk of requiring reintubation or tracheostomy, and posthospital functional disability and quality of life. By closely attending to the mechanisms of respiratory muscle injury and limb muscle injury during mechanical ventilation, ICU clinicians may be able to prevent this injury and improve outcomes for their patients.

The mechanisms responsible for respiratory muscle injury and limb muscle injury are similar, although the timing and severity of their effects differ between the 2 muscle groups; respiratory muscle weakness and limb muscle weakness generally represent 2 independent phenomena, particularly during the early course of mechanical ventilation. Key mechanisms include excessive unloading, excessive concentric or eccentric loading, sepsis and inflammation, and metabolic derangements associated with critical illness.

To prevent the development of muscle weakness, clinicians should strive to mobilize patients as early as possible while paying close attention to mechanical ventilator settings to achieve an optimal level of diaphragm loading (thought to be similar to that of healthy subjects breathing at rest). A range of potential rehabilitative and pharmacologic strategies for preventing and treating respiratory muscle weakness await further investigation. As the field moves to place greater emphasis on improving long-term patient-centered outcomes in ICU survivors, efforts to prevent respiratory and limb muscle weakness will require greater attention from both researchers and clinicians.

REFERENCES

1. Esteban A, Frutos-Vivar F, Muriel A, et al. Evolution of mortality over time in patients receiving mechanical ventilation. Am J Respir Crit Care Med 2013;188(2): 220–30.
2. Doorduin J, Van Hees HWH, Van Der Hoeven JG, et al. Monitoring of the respiratory muscles in the critically ill. Am J Respir Crit Care Med 2013;187(1):20–7.
3. Dres M, Goligher EC, Heunks LMA, et al. Critical illness-associated diaphragm weakness. Intensive Care Med 2017. https://doi.org/10.1007/s00134-017-4928-4.
4. Fan E, Cheek F, Chlan L, et al. An official American Thoracic Society Clinical Practice Guideline: the diagnosis of intensive care unit-acquired weakness in adults. Am J Respir Crit Care Med 2014;190(12):1437–46.
5. Stevens RD, Marshall SA, Cornblath DR, et al. A framework for diagnosing and classifying intensive care unit-acquired weakness. Crit Care Med 2009; 37(Suppl. 10):299–308.
6. Demoule A, Molinari N, Jung B, et al. Patterns of diaphragm function in critically ill patients receiving prolonged mechanical ventilation: a prospective longitudinal study. Ann Intensive Care 2016;6(1):75.
7. Demoule A, Jung B, Prodanovic H, et al. Diaphragm dysfunction on admission to the intensive care unit. prevalence, risk factors, and prognostic impact—a prospective study. Am J Respir Crit Care Med 2013;188(2):213–9.
8. Dres M, Dube BP, Mayaux J, et al. Coexistence and impact of limb muscle and diaphragm weakness at time of liberation from mechanical ventilation in medical intensive care unit patients. Am J Respir Crit Care Med 2017;195(1):57–66.
9. Laghi F, Cattapan SE, Jubran A, et al. Is weaning failure caused by low-frequency fatigue of the diaphragm? Am J Respir Crit Care Med 2003;167: 120–7.
10. Jung B, Moury PH, Mahul M, et al. Diaphragmatic dysfunction in patients with ICU-acquired weakness and its impact on extubation failure. Intensive Care Med 2016;42(5):853–61.
11. Kim WY, Suh HJ, Hong SB, et al. Diaphragm dysfunction assessed by ultrasonography: influence on weaning from mechanical ventilation. Crit Care Med 2011;39(12):2627–30.
12. Ferrari G, De Filippi G, Elia F, et al. Diaphragm ultrasound as a new index of discontinuation from mechanical ventilation. Crit Ultrasound J 2014;6(1). https://doi.org/10.1186/2036-7902-6-8.
13. Jiang JR, Tsai TH, Jerng JS, et al. Ultrasonographic evaluation of liver/spleen movements and extubation outcome. Chest 2004;126(1):179–85.

14. Hooijman PE, Beishuizen A, Witt CC, et al. Diaphragm muscle fiber weakness and ubiquitin-proteasome activation in critically ill patients. Am J Respir Crit Care Med 2015;191(10):1126–38.

15. Van den Berg M, Hooijman PE, Beishuizen A, et al. Diaphragm atrophy and weakness in the absence of mitochondrial dysfunction in the critically ill. Am J Respir Crit Care Med 2017;196(12):1544–58.

16. Levine S, Nguyen T, Taylor N, et al. Rapid disuse atrophy of diaphragm fibers in mechanically ventilated humans. N Engl J Med 2008;358(13):1327–35.

17. Laghi F, Shaikh HS, Morales D, et al. Diaphragmatic neuromechanical coupling and mechanisms of hypercapnia during inspiratory loading. Respir Physiol Neurobiol 2014;198(1):32–41.

18. De Jonghe B, Bastuji-Garin S, Durand M-C, et al. Respiratory weakness is associated with limb weakness and delayed weaning in critical illness. Crit Care Med 2007;35(9):2007–15.

19. De Jonghe B, Sharshar T, Lefaucheur J, et al. Paresis acquired in the intensive care unit. JAMA 2002;288(22):2859–67.

20. Hermans G, Van Mechelen H, Clerckx B, et al. Acute outcomes and 1-year mortality of intensive care unit-acquired weakness: a cohort study and propensity-matched analysis. Am J Respir Crit Care Med 2014;190(4):410–20.

21. Leijten F, Harinck-de Weerd JE, Poortvliet DC, et al. The role of polyneuropathy in motor convalescence after prolonged mechanical ventilation. JAMA 1995;274(15):1221–5.

22. Garnacho-Montero J, Madrazo-Osuna J, García-Garmendia J, et al. Critical illness polyneuropathy: risk factors and clinical consequences. A cohort study in septic patients. Intensive Care Med 2001;27(8):1288–96.

23. Puthucheary ZA, Rawal J, Mcphail M, et al. Acute skeletal muscle wasting in critical illness. JAMA 2013;310(15):1591–600.

24. Schepens T, Verbrugghe W, Dams K, et al. The course of diaphragm atrophy in ventilated patients assessed with ultrasound: a longitudinal cohort study. Crit Care 2015;1–8. https://doi.org/10.1186/s13054-015-1141-0.

25. Goligher EC, Fan E, Herridge MS, et al. Evolution of diaphragm thickness during mechanical ventilation: impact of inspiratory effort. Am J Respir Crit Care Med 2015;192(9):1080–8.

26. Supinski GS, Ann Callahan L. Diaphragm weakness in mechanically ventilated critically ill patients. Crit Care 2013;17(3):R120.

27. Adler D, Dupuis-Lozeron E, Richard J-C, et al. Does inspiratory muscle dysfunction predict readmission after intensive care unit discharge? Am J Respir Crit Care Med 2014;190(3):347–9.

28. Medrinal C, Prieur G, Frenoy É, et al. Respiratory weakness after mechanical ventilation is associated with one-year mortality - a prospective study. Crit Care 2016;20(1):1–7.

29. Goligher EC, Dres M, Fan E, et al. Mechanical ventilation–induced diaphragm atrophy strongly impacts clinical outcomes. Am J Respir Crit Care Med 2018;197(2):204–13.

30. Dos Santos C, Hussain SNA, Mathur S, et al. Mechanisms of chronic muscle wasting and dysfunction after an intensive care unit stay: a pilot study. Am J Respir Crit Care Med 2016;194(7):821–30.

31. Herridge MS, Chu LM, Matte A, et al. The RECOVER program: disability risk groups and 1-year outcome after 7 or more days of mechanical ventilation. Am J Respir Crit Care Med 2016;194(7):831–44.

32. Fan E, Dowdy DW, Colantuoni E, et al. Physical complications in acute lung injury survivors: a 2-year longitudinal prospective study. Crit Care Med 2014; 42(4):849–59.

33. Bolton CF, Gilbert JJ, Hahn AF, et al. Polyneuropathy in critically ill patients. J Neurol Neurosurg Psychiatry 1984;47:1223–31.

34. Kress JP, Hall JB. ICU-acquired weakness and recovery from critical illness. N Engl J Med 2014;370(17):1626–35.

35. Bolton CF. Neuromuscular manifestations of critical illness. Muscle Nerve 2005; 32(2):140–63.

36. Asher RAJ. Dangers of going to bed. Br Med J 1947;2(4536):967–8.

37. Tesch PA, Lundberg TR, Fernandez-Gonzalo R. Unilateral lower limb suspension: from subject selection to "omic" responses. J Appl Physiol 2016;120(10): 1207–14.

38. Jaber S, Jung B, Matecki S, et al. Clinical review: ventilator-induced diaphragmatic dysfunction - human studies confirm animal model findings! Crit Care 2011;15(2):206.

39. Ottenheijm CAC, Van Hees HWH, Heunks LMA, et al. Titin-based mechanosensing and signaling: role in diaphragm atrophy during unloading? Am J Physiol Lung Cell Mol Physiol 2011;300:L161–6.

40. Picard M, Jung B, Liang F, et al. Mitochondrial dysfunction and lipid accumulation in the human diaphragm during mechanical ventilation. Am J Respir Crit Care Med 2012;186(11):1140–9.

41. Powers SK, Shanely RA, Coombes JS, et al. Mechanical ventilation results in progressive contractile dysfunction in the diaphragm. J Appl Physiol 2002;92: 1851–8.

42. Le Bourdelles G, Viires N, Boczkowski J, et al. Effects of mechanical ventilation on diaphragmatic contractile properties in rats. Am J Respir Crit Care Med 1994;149(6):1539–44.

43. Sassoon CSH, Caiozzo VJ, Manka A, et al. Altered diaphragm contractile properties with controlled mechanical ventilation. J Appl Physiol 2002;92(6): 2585–95.

44. Yang L, Luo J, Bourdon J, et al. Controlled mechanical ventilation leads to remodeling of the rat diaphragm. Am J Respir Crit Care Med 2002;166(8): 1135–40.

45. Anzueto A, Peters JI, Tobin MJ, et al. Effects of prolonged controlled mechanical ventilation on diaphragmatic function in healthy adult baboons. Crit Care Med 1997;25(7):1187–90.

46. Radell PJ, Remahl S, Nichols DG, et al. Effects of prolonged mechanical ventilation and inactivity on piglet diaphragm function. Intensive Care Med 2002; 28(3):358–64.

47. Jaber S, Petrof BJ, Jung B, et al. Rapidly progressive diaphragmatic weakness and injury during mechanical ventilation in humans. Am J Respir Crit Care Med 2011;183(3):364–71.

48. Hooijman PE, Beishuizen A, de Waard MC, et al. Diaphragm fiber strength is reduced in critically ill patients and restored by a troponin activator. Am J Respir Crit Care Med 2014;189(7):863–5.

49. Zambon M, Beccaria P, Matsuno J, et al. Mechanical ventilation and diaphragmatic atrophy in critically ill patients: an ultrasound study. Crit Care Med 2016; 44(7):1347–52.

50. Goligher EC, Laghi F, Detsky ME, et al. Measuring diaphragm thickness with ultrasound in mechanically ventilated patients: feasibility, reproducibility and validity. Intensive Care Med 2015. https://doi.org/10.1007/s00134-015-3687-3.
51. Puthucheary Z, Harridge S, Hart N. Skeletal muscle dysfunction in critical care: wasting, weakness, and rehabilitation strategies. Crit Care Med 2010;38(10): 676–82.
52. Jiang T, Reid WD, Road JD. Delayed diaphragm injury and diaphragm force production. Crit Care Med 1998;157:736–42.
53. Reid WD, Huang J, Bryson S, et al. Diaphragm injury and myofibrillar structure induced by resistive loading. J Appl Physiol 1994;76(1):176–84.
54. Laghi F, D'Alfonso N, Tobin MJ. Pattern of recovery from diaphragmatic fatigue over 24 hours. J Appl Physiol 1995;79(2):539–46.
55. Lin MC, Ebihara S, Dwairi QEL, et al. Diaphragm sarcolemmal injury is induced by sepsis and alleviated by nitric oxide synthase inhibition. Am J Respir Crit Care Med 1998;158(5 pt I):1656–63.
56. Ebihara S, Hussain SNA, Danialou G, et al. Mechanical ventilation protects against diaphragm injury in sepsis: interaction of oxidative and mechanical stresses. Am J Respir Crit Care Med 2002;165(2):221–8.
57. Orozco-levi M, Lloreta J, Minguella J, et al. Injury of the human diaphragm associated with exertion and chronic obstructive pulmonary disease. Am J Respir Crit Care Med 2001;164:1734–9.
58. Damas F, Phillips SM, Lixandrão ME, et al. Early resistance training-induced increases in muscle cross-sectional area are concomitant with edema-induced muscle swelling. Eur J Appl Physiol 2016;116(1):49–56.
59. Proske U, Morgan DL. Muscle damage from eccentric exercise: mechanism, mechanical signs, adaptations and clinical applications. J Physiol 2001; 537(2):333–45.
60. Topulos GP, Reid MB, Leith DE. Pliometric activity of inspiratory muscles: maximal pressure-flow curves. J Appl Physiol 1987;62(1):322–7.
61. Gea J, Zhu E, Galdiz JB, et al. Functional consequences of eccentric contractions of the diaphragm. Arch Bronconeumol 2009;45(2):68–74 [in Spanish].
62. Sieck GC, Ferreira LF, Reid MB, et al. Mechanical properties of respiratory muscles. Compr Physiol 2013;3(4):1553–67.
63. Baydur A. Decay of inspiratory muscle pressure during expiration in anesthetized kyphoscoliosis patients. J Appl Physiol 1992;72(2):712–20.
64. Pellegrini M, Hedenstierna G, Roneus A, et al. The diaphragm acts as a brake during expiration to prevent lung collapse. Am J Respir Crit Care Med 2017; 195(12):1608–16.
65. Thille AW, Rodriguez P, Cabello B, et al. Patient-ventilator asynchrony during assisted mechanical ventilation. Intensive Care Med 2006;32(10):1515–22.
66. Akoumianaki E, Lyazidi A, Rey N, et al. Mechanical ventilation-induced reverse-triggered breaths a frequently unrecognized form of neuromechanical coupling. Chest 2013;143(4):927–38.
67. Boczkowski J, Lanone S, Ungureanu-Longrois D, et al. Induction of diaphragmatic nitric oxide synthase after endotoxin administration in rats: role on diaphragmatic contractile dysfunction. J Clin Invest 1996;98(7):1550–9.
68. Supinski GS, Wang W, Callahan LA. Caspase and calpain activation both contribute to sepsis-induced diaphragmatic weakness. J Appl Physiol 2009; 107(5):1389–96.
69. Laghi F, Tobin MJ. State of the art disorders of the respiratory muscles. Am J Respir Crit Care Med 2003;168:10–48.

70. Hermans G, Agten A, Testelmans D, et al. Increased duration of mechanical ventilation is associated with decreased diaphragmatic force: a prospective observational study. Crit Care 2010;14(4). https://doi.org/10.1186/cc9094.

71. Testelmans D, Maes K, Wouters P, et al. Infusions of rocuronium and cisatracurium exert different effects on rat diaphragm function. Intensive Care Med 2007; 33(5):872–9.

72. Papazian L, Forel J-M, Gacouin A, et al. Neuromuscular blockers in early acute respiratory distress syndrome. N Engl J Med 2010;363(12):1107–16.

73. Schakman O, Gilson H, Thissen JP. Mechanisms of glucocorticoid-induced myopathy. J Endocrinol 2008;197(1):1–10.

74. Maes K, Agten A, Smuder A, et al. Corticosteroid effects on ventilator-induced diaphragm dysfunction in anesthetized rats depend on the dose administered. Respir Res 2010;11(1):178.

75. Michelet P, Carreira S, Demoule A, et al. Effects of acute respiratory and metabolic acidosis on diaphragm muscle obtained from rats. Anesthesiology 2015; 122(4):876–83.

76. Schellekens WJM, van Hees HWH, Kox M, et al. Hypercapnia attenuates ventilator-induced diaphragm atrophy and modulates dysfunction. Crit Care 2014;18(1):1–9.

77. Jung B, Sebbane M, Goff CL, et al. Moderate and prolonged hypercapnic acidosis may protect against ventilator-induced diaphragmatic dysfunction in healthy piglet: an in vivo study. Crit Care 2013;17(1):1–8.

78. Callahan L, Supinski GS. Hyperglycemia and acquired weakness in critically ill patients: potential mechanisms. Crit Care 2009;13(2):125.

79. Lewis MI, Feinberg AT, Fournier M. IGF-I and/or growth hormone preserve diaphragm fiber size with moderate malnutrition. J Appl Physiol 1998;85(1):189–97.

80. Barr J, Fraser GL, Puntillo K, et al. Clinical practice guidelines for the management of pain, agitation, and delirium in adult patients in the intensive care unit. Crit Care Med 2013;263–306. https://doi.org/10.1097/CCM.0b013e3182783b72.

81. Bailey P, Thomsen GE, Spuhler VJ, et al. Early activity is feasible and safe in respiratory failure patients. Crit Care Med 2007;35(1):139–45.

82. Turner DA, Cheifetz IM, Rehder KJ, et al. Active rehabilitation and physical therapy during extracorporeal membrane oxygenation while awaiting lung transplantation: a practical approach. Crit Care Med 2011;39(12):2593–8.

83. Griffiths RD, Palmer TE, Helliwell T, et al. Effect of passive stretching on the wasting of muscle in the critically ill. Nutrition 1995;11(5):428–32.

84. Schweickert WD, Pohlman MC, Pohlman AS, et al. Early physical and occupational therapy in mechanically ventilated, critically ill patients: a randomised controlled trial. Lancet 2009;373(9678):1874–82.

85. Denehy L, Skinner EH, Edbrooke L, et al. Exercise rehabilitation for patients with critical illness: a randomized controlled trial with 12 months of follow-up. Crit Care 2013;17(4):R156.

86. Morris PE, Berry MJ, Files DC, et al. Standardized rehabilitation and hospital length of stay among patients with acute respiratory failure a randomized clinical trial. JAMA 2016;315(24):2694–702.

87. Moss M, Nordon-craft A, Malone D, et al. A randomized trial of an intensive physical therapy program for patients with acute respiratory failure. Am J Respir Crit Care Med 2016;193:1101–10.

88. Schaller SJ, Anstey M, Blobner M, et al. Early, goal-directed mobilisation in the surgical intensive care unit: a randomised controlled trial. Lancet 2016; 388(10052):1377–88.
89. Tipping CJ, Harrold M, Holland A, et al. The effects of active mobilisation and rehabilitation in ICU on mortality and function: a systematic review. Intensive Care Med 2017;43(2):171–83.
90. Jung B, Constantin J-M, Rossel N, et al. Adaptive support ventilation prevents ventilator-induced diaphragmatic dysfunction in piglet an in vivo and in vitro study. Anesthesiology 2010;6:1435–43.
91. Mauri T, Grasselli G, Suriano G, et al. Control of respiratory drive and effort in extracorporeal severe acute respiratory distress syndrome. Crit Care Med 2016;125:159–67.
92. Doorduin J, Nollet JL, Roesthuis LH, et al. Partial neuromuscular blockade during partial ventilatory support in sedated patients with high tidal volumes. Am J Respir Crit Care Med 2017;195(8):1033–42.
93. Karagiannidis C, Lubnoow M, Philipp A, et al. Autoregulation of ventilation with neurally adjusted ventilatory assist on extracorporeal lung support. Intensive Care Med 2010;36:2038–44.
94. Elkins M, Dentice R. Inspiratory muscle training facilitates weaning from mechanical ventilation among patients in the intensive care unit: a systematic review. J Physiother 2015;61(3):125–34.
95. Romer LM, McConnell AK. Specificity and reversibility of inspiratory muscle training. Med Sci Sports Exerc 2003;35:237–44.
96. Ayas NT, Cool FDMC, Gore R, et al. Prevention of human diaphragm atrophy with short periods of electrical stimulation. Am J Respir Crit Care Med 1999; 159:2018–20.
97. Martin AD, Joseph AM, Beaver TM, et al. Effect of intermittent phrenic nerve stimulation during cardiothoracic surgery on mitochondrial respiration in the human diaphragm. Crit Care Med 2014;42(2):e152–156.
98. Ahn B, Beaver T, Tomas M, et al. Phrenic nerve stimulation increases human diaphragm fiber force after cardiothoracic surgery. Am J Respir Crit Care Med 2014;190(7):837–9.
99. Reynolds SC, Meyyappan R, Thakkar V, et al. Mitigation of ventilator-induced diaphragm atrophy by transvenous phrenic nerve stimulation. Am J Respir Crit Care Med 2017;195(3):339–48.
100. Reynolds S, Ebner A, Meffen T, et al. Diaphragm activation in ventilated patients using a novel transvenous phrenic nerve pacing catheter. Crit Care Med 2017; 45(7):e691–4.
101. Gibson JN, Smith K, Rennie MJ. Prevention of disuse muscle atrophy by means of electrical stimulation: maintenance of protein synthesis. Lancet 1988;2(8614): 767–70.
102. Jolley SE, Bunnell AE, Hough CL. ICU-acquired weakness. Chest 2016;150(5): 1129–40.
103. Segers J, Hermans G, Bruyninckx F, et al. Feasibility of neuromuscular electrical stimulation in critically ill patients. J Crit Care 2014;29(6):1082–8.
104. Hermans G, Casaer MP, Clerckx B, et al. Effect of tolerating macronutrient deficit on the development of intensive-care unit acquired weakness: a subanalysis of the EPaNIC trial. Lancet Respir Med 2013;1:621–9.
105. Powers SK, Hudson MB, Nelson WB, et al. Mitochondrial-targeted antioxidants protect against mechanical ventilation-induced diaphragm weakness. Crit Care Med 2011;39(7):1749–59.

106. Agten A, Maes K, Smuder A, et al. N-Acetylcysteine protects the rat diaphragm from the decreased contractility associated with controlled mechanical ventilation. Crit Care Med 2011;39(4):777–82.

107. Travaline JM, Sudarshan S, Roy BG, et al. Effect of N -acetylcysteine on human diaphragm strength and fatigability. Am J Respir Crit Care Med 1997;156: 1567–71.

108. Takala J, Ruokonen E, Webster NR, et al. Increased mortality associated with growth hormone treatment in critically ill adults. N Engl J Med 1999;341:785–92.

109. Schols AMWJ, Soeters PB, Mostert ROB. Physiologic effects of nutritional support and anabolic steroids in patients with chronic obstructive pulmonary disease. Am J Respir Crit Care Med 1995;152:1268–74.

110. Almoosa KF, Gupta A, Pedroza C, et al. Low testosterone levels are frequent in patients with acute respiratory failure and are associated with poor outcomes. Endocr Pract 2014;20(10):1057–63.

111. Kim WY, Park SH, Kim WY, et al. Effect of theophylline on ventilator-induced diaphragmatic dysfunction. J Crit Care 2016;33:145–50.

112. Doorduin J, Sinderby CA, Beck J, et al. The calcium sensitizer levosimendan improves human diaphragm function. Am J Respir Crit Care Med 2012;185(1): 90–5.

113. van Hees HWH, Dekhuijzen PNR, Heunks LMA. Levosimendan enhances force generation of diaphragm muscle from patients with chronic obstructive pulmonary disease. Am J Respir Crit Care Med 2009;179:41–7.

114. Boussuges A, Gole Y, Blanc P. Diaphragmatic motion studied by M-mode ultrasonography. Chest 2009;135(2):391–400.

115. Gottesman E, Mccool FD. Ultrasound evaluation of the paralyzed diaphragm. Am J Respir Crit Care Med 1997;155:1570–4.

116. Black LF, Hyatt RE. Maximal respiratory pressures: normal values and relationships to age and sex. Am Rev Respir Dis 1969;99:696–702.

117. Uldry C, Fitting JW. Maximal values of sniff nasal inspiratory pressure in healthy subjects. Thorax 1995;50(4):371–5.

118. Gibson GJ, Whitelaw W, Siafakas N, et al. American Thoracic Society/European Respiratory Society ATS/ERS statement on respiratory muscle testing. Am J Respir Crit Care Med 2002;166:518–624.

119. Watson AC, Hughes PD, Harris ML, et al. Measurement of twitch transdiaphragmatic, esophageal, and endotracheal tube pressure with bilateral anterolateral magnetic phrenic nerve stimulation in patients in the intensive care unit. Crit Care Med 2001;29(7):1325–31.

120. Liu L, Liu H, Yang Y, et al. Neuroventilatory efficiency and extubation readiness in critically ill patients. Crit Care 2012;16(4):R143.

121. Ali NA, O'Brien JMJ, Hoffmann SP, et al. Acquired weakness, handgrip strength, and mortality in critically ill patients. Am J Respir Crit Care Med 2008;178(3): 261–8.

122. Connolly B, Macbean V, Crowley C, et al. Ultrasound for the assessment of peripheral skeletal muscle architecture in critical illness: a systematic review. Crit Care Med 2015;43(4):897–905.

123. Laghi F, Khan N, Schnell T, et al. New device for nonvolitional evaluation of quadriceps force in ventilated patients. Muscle Nerve 2017;1–8. https://doi.org/10.1002/mus.26026.

124. Latronico N, Bolton CF, Care N. Critical illness polyneuropathy and myopathy: a major cause of muscle weakness and paralysis. Lancet Neurol 2011;10(10): 931–41.

125. Latronico N, Nattino G, Guarneri B, et al. Validation of the peroneal nerve test to diagnose critical illness polyneuropathy and myopathy in the intensive care unit: the multicentre Italian CRIMYNE-2 diagnostic accuracy study. F1000Res 2014. https://doi.org/10.12688/f1000research.3933.1.
126. Hulzebos EHJ, Helders PJM, Favié NJ, et al. Muscle training to prevent postoperative pulmonary complications in high-risk. JAMA 2006;296(15):1851–7.
127. Latronico N, Herridge M, Hopkins RO, et al. The ICM research agenda on intensive care unit-acquired weakness. Intensive Care Med 2017;43(9):1270–81.

Automation of Mechanical Ventilation

Richard D. Branson, MSc, RRT, FCCM

KEYWORDS

- Intensive care unit • Mechanical ventilation • Closed loop ventilation • Weaning

KEY POINTS

- Mechanical ventilation is ubiquitous to intensive care.
- Mechanical ventilation has the potential for harm and management by experienced clinicians is mandatory.
- Automated control of ventilation may provide some advantages related to consistency of care and maintaining evidenced based protocols.

INTRODUCTION

Mechanical ventilation is ubiquitous to intensive care. In fact, the foundation of intensive care units (ICUs) can be traced to housing patients requiring mechanical ventilation for specialized care. In the past 2 decades, our understanding of mechanical ventilation and its complications has become steeped in evidence and physiology. After nearly 60 years of modern positive pressure ventilation, it seems that mechanical ventilation has a fairly narrow therapeutic index between the effective and lethal dose. Clearly, the impact of tidal volume (V_T) and airway pressures on ventilator-induced lung injury and mortality are firmly established.[1]

Yet, even in the presence of evidenced-based guidelines,[2] clinicians routinely ignore even the best proven strategies.[3] The complexity of mechanical ventilation and of ventilators has done little to improve this reality. Clinicians are influenced by local champions, manufacturers, and mentors. This is frequently manifest in the way individuals describe ventilation techniques by the proprietary names of devices, versus by function. In the face of this conundrum, the failure of trained clinicians to adopt evidence-based practices, automation of ventilation settings could provide a solution. However, this remains to be proven. This article reviews the evidence regarding the use of automated control of mechanical ventilation.

Division of Trauma and Critical Care, University of Cincinnati, 231 Albert Sabin Way #558, Cincinnati, OH 45267, USA
E-mail address: Richard.branson@uc.edu

Crit Care Clin 34 (2018) 383–394
https://doi.org/10.1016/j.ccc.2018.03.012
0749-0704/18/© 2018 Elsevier Inc. All rights reserved.

DEFINITIONS

A closed loop control describes a system that changes its output based on a desired input. These systems are also referred to as feedback control systems. In the most basic forms, closed loop control is part and parcel of every mechanical ventilation system. Pressure support uses the pressure signal as a target and controls flow to reach and maintain the desired pressure. This is accomplished by a rapid initial flow followed by a quickly decelerating flow pattern. Wysocki and colleagues[4] have classified closed loop systems based on the level of sophistication into simple, physiologic signal based, and explicit computerized protocols (ECP). **Table 1** provides examples of these 3 types of closed loop systems.

A simple closed loop system includes pressure support or pressure control ventilation. A physiologic signal-based system would include neurally adjusted ventilatory assist (NAVA) or proportional assist ventilation. In these examples, output is increased or decreased in proportion to the input signal. In the case of NAVA, the pressure applied is proportional to the integral of the electrical activity of the diaphragm. Thus, as patient effort increases and electrical activity of the diaphragm is greater, the level of assistance is greater.[5]

Table 1
Classification of closed loop systems based on sophistication

Control	Example	Output	Input(s)	Comments
Simple	Pressure support ventilation	Flow	Airway pressure	
Physiologic signal based	NAVA	Pressure	EAdi	Delivered instantaneous airway pressure is proportional to the integral of the EAdi. During NAVA, the breath is triggered and cycled based on EAdi. The airway pressure applied by the ventilator is determined as: Airway Pressure = NAVA level × EAdi, where airway pressure (cm H_2O), EAdi is the instantaneous integral of the diaphragmatic electrical activity signal (μV), and the NAVA level (cm $H_2O/\mu V$) is a proportionality constant set by the clinician.
Explicit computerized protocol	SmartCarePS	Pressure	Delivered V_T Respiratory frequency End tidal CO_2	Smart care uses a number of clinician inputs to alter ventilator operation. The range of acceptable ventilation can be altered in the presence of COPD or neurologic injury. Additionally, the choice of 'night rest', prevents weaning during selected overnight hours.

Abbreviations: CO_2, carbon dioxide; COPD, chronic obstructive pulmonary disease; EAdi, electrical activity of the diaphragm; NAVA, neurally adjusted ventilatory assist; V_T, tidal volume.

An ECP is medical knowledge resident in technology, applied to specific decision making for an individual patient at a particular point in time.[4] ECP systems may use multiple inputs to control a single ventilator output (pressure support level in Smart-CarePS) or multiple inputs to control several ventilator outputs as seen with Intellivent adaptive support ventilation (iASV).[6,7] The rules in an ECP can include a series of, "if..., then" statements. For example, during closed loop control of inspired oxygen, "*if* oxygen saturation from pulse oximetry (SpO_2) is less than 90% *then* increase the inspired oxygen concentration (Fio_2) by 0.05." These "if... then" statements can become similar to decision making by clinicians, taking into account the difference between the SpO_2 target and the measured value, the number of hypoxemic events in the last hour and the stability of SpO_2, to alter the interval if Fio_2 adjustment. As an example, if the difference between the actual and target SpO_2 is 10% the adjustment in Fio_2 might be 0.10 every 30 seconds compared with an SpO_2 difference of 2%, resulting in a change in Fio_2 of 0.02 every 30 seconds. During SmartCare PS, the change in pressure support level varies based on the desired respiratory frequency, end-tidal carbon dioxide ($ETCO_2$), and V_T. The range of acceptable values for these variables can be altered by the clinician for a given patient in the setting of chronic obstructive pulmonary disease (COPD) or neurologic injury. In the former, the acceptable $ETCO_2$ is higher, whereas in the latter the range of $ETCO_2$ is lower. In this manner, the ventilator is making decisions based on individual patient characteristics, just as the caregiver might.

Chatburn and associates[8] have proposed a more complex system for describing mechanical ventilator operation during traditional and closed loop control. This classification uses 7 separate terms for describing the targeting schemes for ventilator modes. These include set point, dual, servo, adaptive, biovariable, optimal, and intelligent.[8] Aside from the added complexity, the use of engineering terms, although consistent with the literature, also seems to infer a value judgment. For instance, intelligent implies a system that is, perhaps, superior to optimal. In some ways, however, this is also a system that is based on increasing sophistication. Evidence is required to in fact conclude that intelligent is superior to set-point targeting. In fact, the use of volume control, continuous mandatory ventilation, a set-point targeting scheme is the only method to date that has demonstrated an impact on outcome. That being the control of V_T during ventilator support of acute respiratory distress syndrome.[9]

PROPOSED ADVANTAGES

Closed loop control is thought to offer a number of advantages compared with traditional physician control of mechanical ventilation. The sheer number of physiologic variables available to the bedside clinician is daunting. Coupled with the dozens of clinical decisions that must be made daily, the opportunity for error is significant. Despite our best efforts, the ability of the human mind to deal with this volume of information is limited.[10] Staffing shortages, long hours, and overnight shifts only serve to compound these issues.

The implementation of closed loop control may help to relieve the burden of decisions by maintaining ventilation and oxygenation in prescribed ranges while adhering to lung protective rules.[4] Additional advantages could include reduced costs, provision of appropriate care in remote environments in the absence of experts, reduced practice variation, reduced weaning times, and implementation of evidence-based guidelines.[11]

AUTOMATED CONTROL OF MECHANICAL VENTILATION

Although closed loop control is available in a number of ventilator modes including PSV, PCV, NAVA, proportional assist ventilation, and adaptive pressure control, the emphasis of this article is on the use of automated mechanical ventilation and, specifically, on the ventilation modes that adjust support to meet patient demand during maintenance ventilation and weaning. The techniques to be considered include adaptive support ventilation (ASV), iASV, and SmartCare PS.

ADAPTIVE SUPPORT VENTILATION

ASV is a closed loop mode of mechanical ventilation designed to titrate ventilator output on a breath-by-breath basis. The level of ventilatory support provided by the ventilator is determined by respiratory mechanics and breathing effort. The goal of ASV is to provide a preset level of minute ventilation while minimizing the work of breathing. Under normal conditions, the minute volume setting is set at 100% of a normal minute volume based on predicted body weight of 0.1 L/kg/min. Thus, a 70-kg patient would receive a minute ventilation of 7.0 L/min.

ASV adjusts the inspiratory pressure to achieve a respiratory pattern (V_T and frequency) that minimizes the work of breathing based on the Otis equation. Importantly, however, the range of available V_T is controlled by the maximum pressure setting selected by a clinician. Breaths alternate between pressure control and pressure support breaths based on the presence or absence of spontaneous breathing efforts. Conceptually, ASV can provide synchronized intermittent mandatory ventilation and PSV, but in this author's experience, breaths are either all mandatory or spontaneous. During mandatory breaths, ASV controls the inspiratory time and inspiratory:expiratory ratio (I:E) based on measurement of the expiratory time constant. Lower compliance results in a short I:E, whereas a high resistance results in a longer I:E to avoid air trapping. ASV requires the clinician set Fio_2 and positive end-expiratory pressure (PEEP).

ASV is a rule-based technique that guides the patient to achieve a minimum minute ventilation using an "optimal" breathing pattern. ASV uses "hard" and "soft" rules. Hard rules are preset limits unaffected by user input or patient mechanics. An example of a hard rule is the high-pressure limit. The ventilator will not exceed the pressure limit, despite failure to achieve other preset goals. Soft rules are determined by clinician input and respiratory mechanics. Soft rules generally have a range of operation and may change with time and clinician input. The details of ASV operation have been discussed extensively elsewhere.[12–17]

Clinical Studies of Adaptive Support Ventilation

ASV can be used to provide support during the initiation, maintenance, and weaning of mechanical ventilation. Each of these implementations have been studied in human subjects. These topics are considered separately.

ASV has been used in a number of studies evaluating time to discontinuation of ventilatory support after coronary artery bypass surgery.[18–23,25,26] Studying this large, relatively homogenous, readily available population is attractive on many levels. However, this population requires ventilation primarily as a "casualty of anesthesia" and under normal circumstances have minor lung injury.[27] In these 8 studies, the impact on duration of ventilation favors ASV in 4 instances and demonstrates no difference in 4 instances. **Table 2** describes the studies and outcomes. Of note, these studies find that ASV required fewer clinician/ventilator interventions, fewer arterial blood gases, fewer ventilator alarms, and a lesser incidence of postoperative atelectasis on radiographs.

There are several additional areas of concern with ASV in this environment. The first is related to the concept of automated weaning. To decrease the level of ventilator

Table 2
Clinical studies of ASV after cardiac surgery

First Author	Sample Size	Population	Comparator	Primary Outcome	Findings
Sulzer et al,[18] 2001	36	Uncomplicated fast track cardiac surgery	PSV	Duration of ventilation	ASV shorter duration of ventilation 3.2 h vs 4.1 h; Fewer blood gases in the ASV group; No difference in sedation requirements
Cassina et al,[19] 2003	155	Uncomplicated fast track cardiac surgery	None	Duration of ventilation	Duration of ventilation was 3.6 h; V_T was 8.7 ± 1.4 mL/kg
Petter et al,[20] 2003	34	Uncomplicated "fast track" cardiac surgery	SIMV followed by PSV	Duration of ventilation	No difference in duration of ventilation 2.7 vs 3.2 h; No difference in sedation requirements
Gruber et al,[21] 2008	48	Uncomplicated fast track cardiac surgery	AutoMode, PRVC, and volume support	Duration of ventilation	Shorter duration of ventilation with ASV 300 vs 540 min; No difference in number of blood gases or ventilator manipulations
Dongelmans et al,[22] 2009	121	Non–fast track coronary bypass surgery	PCV followed by PSV	Duration of ventilation	No difference in duration of ventilation 16.4 h vs 16.3 h; No difference in sedation requirements
Dongelmans et al,[23] 2010	126	Non–fast track coronary bypass surgery	ASV	Duration of ventilation	No difference in the duration of ventilation 10.8 h vs 10.7 h
Zhu et al,[24] 2015	53	Uncomplicated fast track cardiac valvular surgery	SIMV or SIMV + PSV	Duration of ventilation	Shorter duration of ventilation with ASV 205 min vs 342 min
Tam et al,[25] 2016	52	Uncomplicated fast track cardiac surgery	ASV at a constant V_E target vs ASV with a decremental V_E target	Duration of ventilation	Shorter duration of ventilation with decremental ASV 145 min vs 309 min; No difference in adverse events
Moradian et al,[26] 2017	115	Uncomplicated fast track cardiac surgery	ASV vs SIMV + PSV	Duration of ventilation	No difference in duration of ventilation; Fewer alarms and caregiver interactions with ASV

Abbreviations: ASV, adaptive support ventilation; PCV, pressure control ventilation; PRVC, pressure regulated volume control; PSV, pressure support ventilation; SIMV, synchronized intermittent mandatory ventilation; V_E, minute ventilation; V_T, tidal volume.

assistance, the clinician must decrease the target minute volume. This approach seems to facilitate faster ventilator discontinuation. However, the requirement for clinician intervention, adds an "open loop" to the closed loop system. Choosing the appropriate minute volume target has not been extensively studied and requires some elucidation.[25,28,29] The selected V_T during ASV can exceed lung protective limits and the potential for ventilator-induced lung injury after surgery is a concern.[30]

Several recent trials have evaluated ASV for weaning in patients with acute respiratory failure. Chen and colleagues[31] reported their experience with ASV in a 16-bed Chinese ICU staffed by a single respiratory therapist during the day and no coverage at night. They compared the management of patients with ASV with a matched historical control using synchronized intermittent mandatory ventilation and PSV. Under these rather unique circumstances, the authors demonstrated that patients in the ASV group achieved extubation readiness within 1 day of enrollment more often, achieved weaning within 21 days. However, there were no differences in the duration of ICU or hospital stay. These findings must be considered in light of this unique staffing model. However, a potential advantage of closed loop ventilation is the ability to continue care in the absence or unavailability of caregivers. This study seems to support this thesis.

Kirakli and colleagues[32] compared ASV with PSV for weaning in patients with COPD. They found that patients ventilated with ASV had shorter weaning times and equivalent weaning success. However, the total duration of ventilatory support did not change. The use of ASV for weaning after recovery from acute respiratory failure and after liver transplantation has been reported.[31,33]

ASV has been used successfully as a primary mode of ventilator support during acute respiratory failure. The algorithm based on an expiratory time constant was shown to set I:E and respiratory frequency appropriately for both obstructive and restrictive disease. These reports find a reduction in manual ventilator adjustments, similar gas exchange, and perhaps improved CO_2 elimination for a given combination of V_T and respiratory frequency.[34–36] Patients with obstructive disease in these trials, however, can receive V_Ts outside suggested lung protective values.

One criticism of ASV has been the finding that the V_T may approach 9 to 10 mL/kg in some patients.[30,37–39] This limitation can be overcome by appropriate setting of the maximum pressure and V_T limits. ASV has been commercially available for more than 20 years and widespread adoption has not occurred. Although ASV may facilitate weaning when the percent of minute volume value is appropriately set, it seems to have no clear advantage over manual techniques. Closed loop techniques can decrease practice variation through appropriate selection of hard rules, such a maximum pressure chosen by the operator. This author has previously argued that techniques like ASV may provide the greatest benefit in resource-limited environments, and the work by Chen and colleagues[31] seems to support this opinion.

Intellivent Adaptive Support Ventilation

Intellivent ASV is the logical extension of ASV to include the automated selection of Fio_2 and PEEP. The PEEP/Fio_2 controller uses the PEEP tables from the ARDS Network's prospective randomized multicenter trial of 6 mL/kg versus 12 mL/kg V_T for the treatment of acute lung injury and acute respiratory distress syndrome (ARMA) and the ARDS Network's prospective multi-center trial of higher end-expiratory lung volume/lower Fio_2 versus lower end-expiratory lung volume/ higher Fio_2 ventilation in acute lung injury and acute respiratory distress syndrome (ALVEOLI).[38] The ARMA trial used an aggressive Fio_2 strategy, whereas the ALVEOLI trial is PEEP intensive. An integral pulse oximeter provides the input signal to the ventilator, where the clinician can set the desired SpO_2. Pulse volume variability from the oximeter can also provide information regarding patient hemodynamic status, limiting the use of PEEP in favor of Fio_2 during hemodynamic compromise. Intellivent is currently not commercially available in the United States.

The minimum PEEP is 5 cm H_2O, and at initiation the controller uses the ARMA PEEP/Fio_2 table to reach the desired SpO_2. After stabilization the Fio_2 and PEEP, patients are weaned using the ALVEOLI table. **Fig. 1** provides a pictograph of the PEEP/Fio_2 tables used during Intellivent.

Clinical studies of Intellivent adaptive support ventilation

The use of iASV has been limited owing to the recent introduction and unavailability in the United States. In a preliminary trial of sedated patients with acute respiratory failure, Arnal and colleagues[7] demonstrated that, during a 2-hour crossover trial, iASV provided ventilation at a lower airway pressure, volume, and Fio_2 while producing the same results in terms of oxygenation compared with ASV. The V_TS were slightly lower with iASV and $Paco_2$ higher. In a follow-up crossover trial, iASV applied for 24 hours compared with PSV demonstrated improved oxygenation. In this study, PEEP was higher and more variable during iASV, as might be expected.[40] The authors suggest that the biovariability of PEEP might explain the improved oxygenation.

Arnal and colleagues applied iASV in a wide range of patient populations ventilated for less than 24 hours and found that ventilator settings were selected appropriately based on the lung condition, particularly in passive patients. However, like traditional ASV, spontaneously breathing subjects (breathing with adaptive pressure support) have less variability in volume and pattern.[41] A randomized trial

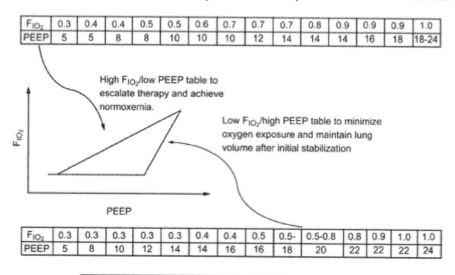

Fig. 1. Combination of the positive end-expiratory pressure (PEEP)–fraction of inspired oxygen (FIO$_2$) tables from the ARDSnet ARMA and ARDSnet ALVEOLI trials used for increasing and decreasing oxygenation support during Intellivent adaptive support ventilation (iASV). SpO$_2$, oxygen saturation. (*From* Branson RD. Modes to facilitate ventilator weaning. Respir Care 2012;57:1642; with permission.)

of iASV compared safety and efficacy with modes chosen by the attending physician as the time spent within previously defined ranges of nonoptimal and optimal ventilation. Interestingly, iASV was more likely to be in the suboptimal range for maximum pressure. As in previous trials, iASV made more manipulations but required fewer clinician interactions and the variability of volumes and airway pressures were greater.[42]

Fot and colleagues[43] evaluated iASV compared with protocolized weaning and synchronized intermittent mandatory ventilation plus PSV after coronary bypass grafting. They found that iASV and protocolized weaning had similar outcomes and shortened weaning compared with traditional methods. The authors noted the decrease in clinician interactions with the ventilator, but no other advantages. More recently, Arnal and associates compared iASV with either PSV or volume control, continuous mandatory ventilation in 60 subjects. They concluded that iASV decreases the number of manual ventilator setting changes with no difference in the number of arterial blood gas analyses or sedation use. Using a Likert scale, caregivers rated iASV as easier to use compared with conventional ventilation modes.[44]

SmartCARE PS

SmartCarePS describes control of PSV where the pressure support level is based on the patient's V_T, respiratory frequency, $ETCO_2$, and a series of preset parameters based on the patient condition (presence of COPD or neurologic injury). SmartCarePS adjusts pressure support to maintain the patient in a "normal" range of ventilation. A normal range of ventilation is typically defined as a V_T of 300 mL, a respiratory frequency between 12 and 30 breaths/min, and an $ETCO_2$ of less than 55 mm Hg (these settings can be adapted for subjects with COPD or neurologic injury). Outside of the normal range, SmartCarePS defines other conditions and manipulates the pressure support based on the current value, the clinician input parameters, and the patient's historical breathing pattern. SmartCarePS is intended for weaning and, therefore, not used clinically for the support of acute respiratory failure.[11]

Clinical studies of SmartCare PS

Introduced in 1996, SmartCare PS has been evaluated in a number of weaning trials.[6,45–51] The original trial simply compared the duration of ventilation in the specified ranges of comfort compared with clinician-selected PSV. This study found that SmartCarePS maintained patients in the desired ranges far more frequently.[45] Lellouche and coworkers[47] published the first and largest randomized trial compared with traditional weaning in 5 European centers in 2006. This report found significantly quicker weaning times with SmartCarePS compared with traditional weaning. However, in at least 2 centers, spontaneous breathing trials were not used in the control arm.[47] This is a limitation of the study, but represents a pragmatic trial. Across the world, the use of protocolized weaning is espoused by clinical practice guidelines[52] but not routinely implemented.

Subsequent trials of SmartCarePS have found both advantages and no advantage compared with traditional weaning based on patient condition (sepsis vs COPD vs cardiac surgery), the type and staffing of the ICU, and patient age (adults vs pediatrics).[48–51] Cochrane reviews of automated weaning routinely find that automated weaning demonstrates approximately a 30% reduction in weaning time compared with traditional weaning. However, lack of standards in the control arm of trials, heterogeneity, and small numbers limit the strength of these conclusions.[53] Large multicenter trials are needed to determine the value of SmartCarePS in routine care.

Concerns with the Automated Control of Ventilation

Automation of mechanical ventilation has a number of advantages, as described. The potential disadvantages are less frequently discussed, but require additional research. As an example, if the ventilation system increases PEEP and or Fio_2 rapidly in response to hypoxemia and prevents the typical desaturation events that routinely alert caregivers to worsening lung function, this event must be communicated to the staff. Increases in PEEP and airway pressures that may result in hemodynamic compromise also require additional safety measures. As clinicians, we consider heart rate, blood pressure, filling pressures, vasopressor therapy, and fluid status during the manipulation of mean airway pressures. At present, no ventilation system has the ability to include these additional inputs into the ventilator decision process. It may be that limiting changes in PEEP to less than 12 cm H_2O is needed and increases beyond this value approved by the clinician with knowledge of hemodynamic performance and current therapy.

As seen with several of these techniques, certain situations can result in excessive V_T and pressure delivery, perhaps leading to ventilator-induced lung injury. Alarm settings and alert settings require additional care.

SUMMARY

Simple closed loop control of mechanical ventilation is routine and operates behind the ventilator interface. More complex systems described as intelligent control or ECP, are commercially available but have yet to gain widespread acceptance.[54] New trials demonstrating a cost benefit of automated ventilation are required. Simply reducing the number of caregiver interactions is neither an advantage for the patient or the staff. In fact, automated systems causing lack of situational awareness of the ICU are a concern. Along with these autonomous systems must come monitoring and displays that easily inform the staff of the patients current condition and response to therapy. Alert notifications for sudden escalation of therapy are required to ensure patient safety.

The use of automated ventilation clearly has utility in remote settings in the absence of experts. There are more than 1000 critical access hospitals in the United States, most with fewer than 50 beds that are the entry point to the health care system in rural America. These hospital lack ICUs and ICU and respiratory care expertise. Remote care in disaster and military medicine is another area where local expertise may not match the severity of patient illness. These environments represent a natural fit for automated ventilation. However, the cost and size of devices require modification.

Whether automated ventilation will be accepted in large academic medical centers remains to be seen. Despite staffing shortages and increased patient acuity, this author has never heard the ICU staff express that the solution to current concerns in the ICU is more automation of ventilator support.

REFERENCES

1. Needham DM, Yang T, Dinglas VD, et al. Timing of low tidal volume ventilation and intensive care unit mortality in acute respiratory distress syndrome. A prospective cohort study. Am J Respir Crit Care Med 2015;191(2):177–85.
2. Fan E, Del Sorbo L, Goligher EC, et al, American Thoracic Society, European Society of Intensive Care Medicine, and Society of Critical Care Medicine. An official American Thoracic Society/European Society of intensive care medicine/Society of Critical Care Medicine clinical practice guideline: mechanical ventilation in

adult patients with acute respiratory distress syndrome. Am J Respir Crit Care Med 2017;195:1253–63.

3. Morris AH. Human cognitive limitations. Broad, consistent, clinical application of physiological principles will require decision support. Ann Am Thorac Soc 2018; 15(Supplement 1):S53–6.

4. Wysocki M, Jouvet P, Jaber S. Closed loop mechanical ventilation. J Clin Monit Comput 2014;28(1):49–56.

5. Sinderby C, Navalesi P, Beck J, et al. Neural control of mechanical ventilation in respiratory failure. Nat Med 1999;5:1433–6.

6. Dojat M, Harf A, Touchard D, et al. Clinical evaluation of a computer-controlled pressure support mode. Am J Respir Crit Care Med 2000;161(4 Pt 1):1161–6.

7. Arnal JM, Wysocki M, Novotni D, et al. Safety and efficacy of a fully closed-loop control ventilation (IntelliVent-ASV®) in sedated ICU patients with acute respiratory failure: a prospective randomized crossover study. Intensive Care Med 2012;38:781–7.

8. Chatburn RL, El-Khatib M, Mireles-Cabodevila E. A taxonomy for mechanical ventilation: 10 fundamental maxims. Respir Care 2014;59:1747–63.

9. Acute Respiratory Distress Syndrome Network. Ventilation with lower tidal volumes as compared with traditional tidal volumes for acute lung injury and the acute respiratory distress syndrome. N Engl J Med 2000;342:1301–8.

10. Miller G. The magical number seven plus or minus two: some limits on our capacity for processing information. Psychol Rev 1956;63:81–97.

11. Branson RD. Modes to facilitate ventilator weaning. Respir Care 2012;57:1635–48.

12. Laubscher TP, Frutiger A, Fanconi S, et al. Automatic selection of tidal volume, respiratory frequency and minute volume in intubated ICU patients as startup procedure for closed-loop controlled ventilation. Int J Clin Monit Comput 1994; 11:19–30.

13. Laubscher TP, Frutiger A, Fanconi S, et al. The automatic selection of ventilation parameters during the initial phase of mechanical ventilation. Intensive Care Med 1996;22:199–207.

14. Branson RD, Campbell RS, Davis K, et al. Closed loop ventilation. Respir Care 2002;47:427–53.

15. Johannigman JA, Barnes SA, Muskat P, et al. Autonomous control of ventilation. J Trauma 2008;64(4 Suppl):S302–20.

16. Campbell RS, Branson RD, Johannigman JA. Adaptive support ventilation. Respir Care Clin N Am 2001;7(3):425–40.

17. Brunner JX, Iotti GA. Adaptive support ventilation (ASV). Minerva Anestesiol 2002;68(5):365–8.

18. Sulzer CF, Chiolero R, Chassot PG, et al. Adaptive support ventilation for fast tracheal extubation after cardiac surgery: a randomized controlled study. Anesthesiology 2001;95:1339–45.

19. Cassina T, Chiolero R, Mauri R, et al. Clinical experience with adaptive support ventilation for fast-track cardiac surgery. J Cardiothorac Vasc Anesth 2003;17: 571–5.

20. Petter AH, Chioléro RL, Cassina T, et al. Automatic "respirator/weaning" with adaptive support ventilation: the effect on duration of endotracheal intubation and patient management. Anesth Analg 2003;97:1743–50.

21. Gruber PC, Gomersall CD, Leung P, et al. Randomized controlled trial comparing adaptive-support ventilation with pressure-regulated volume-controlled ventilation with automode in weaning patients after cardiac surgery. Anesthesiology 2008;109:81–7.

22. Dongelmans DA, Veelo DP, Paulus F, et al. Weaning automation with adaptive support ventilation: a randomized controlled trial in cardiothoracic surgery patients. Anesth Analg 2009;108:565–71.

23. Dongelmans DA, Veelo DP, Binnekade JM, et al. Adaptive support ventilation with protocolized de-escalation and escalation does not accelerate tracheal extubation of patients after nonfast-track cardiothoracic surgery. Anesth Analg 2010; 111(4):961–7.

24. Zhu F, Gomersall CD, Ng SK, et al. A randomized controlled trial of adaptive support ventilation mode to wean patients after fast-track cardiac valvular surgery. Anesthesiology 2015;122(4):832–40.

25. Tam MK, Wong WT, Gomersall CD, et al. A randomized controlled trial of 2 protocols for weaning cardiac surgical patients receiving adaptive support ventilation. J Crit Care 2016;33:163–8.

26. Moradian ST, Saeid Y, Ebadi A, et al. Adaptive support ventilation reduces the incidence of atelectasis in patients undergoing coronary artery bypass grafting: a randomized clinical trial. Anesth Pain Med 2017;7(3):e44619.

27. Esquinas AM, Cravo J, De Santo LS. Adaptive support ventilation weaning protocols in cardiac surgical patients: complex speculations with little practical impact. J Crit Care 2017;37:250.

28. Kiaei BA, Kashefi P, Hashemi ST, et al. The comparison effects of two methods of (adaptive support ventilation minute ventilation: 110% and adaptive support ventilation minute ventilation: 120%) on mechanical ventilation and hemodynamic changes and length of being in recovery in intensive care units. Adv Biomed Res 2017;6:52.

29. Wu CP, Lin HI, Perng WC, et al. Correlation between the %MinVol setting and work of breathing during adaptive support ventilation in patients with respiratory failure. Respir Care 2010;55:334–41.

30. Dongelmans DA, Veelo DP, Bindels A, et al. Determinants of tidal volumes with adaptive support ventilation: a multicenter observational study. Anesth Analg 2008;107:932–7.

31. Chen CW, Wu CP, Dai YL, et al. Effects of implementing adaptive support ventilation in a medical intensive care unit. Respir Care 2011;56:976–83.

32. Kirakli C, Ozdemir I, Ucar ZZ, et al. Adaptive support ventilation for faster weaning in COPD: a randomised controlled trial. Eur Respir J 2011;38:774–80.

33. Celli P, Privato E, Ianni S, et al. Adaptive support ventilation versus synchronized intermittent mandatory ventilation with pressure support in weaning patients after orthotopic liver transplantation. Transplant Proc 2014;46:2272–8.

34. Arnal JM, Wysocki M, Nafati C, et al. Automatic selection of breathing pattern using adaptive support ventilation. Intensive Care Med 2008;34:75–81.

35. Iotti GA, Polito A, Belliato M, et al. Adaptive support ventilation versus conventional ventilation for total ventilatory support in acute respiratory failure. Intensive Care Med 2010;36:1371–9.

36. Agarwal R, Srinivasan A, Aggarwal AN, et al. Adaptive support ventilation for complete ventilatory support in acute respiratory distress syndrome: a pilot, randomized controlled trial. Respirology 2013;18:1108–15.

37. Dongelmans DA, Paulus F, Veelo DP, et al. Adaptive support ventilation may deliver unwanted respiratory rate-tidal volume combinations in patients with acute lung injury ventilated according to an open lung concept. Anesthesiology 2011;114:1138–43.

38. Veelo DP, Dongelmans DA, Binnekade JM, et al. Adaptive support ventilation: a translational study evaluating the size of delivered tidal volumes. Int J Artif Organs 2010;33:302–9.
39. Acute Respiratory Distress Syndrome Network. Higher versus lower positive end-expiratory pressures in patients with acute respiratory distress syndrome. N Engl J Med 2004;351:327–36.
40. Arnal JM, Garnero A, Novonti D, et al. Feasibility study on full closed-loop control ventilation (IntelliVent-ASV™) in ICU patients with acute respiratory failure: a prospective observational comparative study. Crit Care 2013;17(5):R196.
41. Clavieras N, Wysocki M, Coisel Y, et al. Prospective randomized crossover study of a new closed-loop control system versus pressure support during weaning from mechanical ventilation. Anesthesiology 2013;119:631–41.
42. Bialais E, Wittebole X, Vignaux L, et al. Closed-loop ventilation mode (IntelliVent®-ASV) in intensive care unit: a randomized trial. Minerva Anestesiol 2016;82:657–68.
43. Fot EV, Izotova NN, Yudina AS, et al. Automated weaning from mechanical ventilation after off-pump coronary artery bypass grafting. Front Med (Lausanne) 2017;4:31.
44. Arnal JM, Garnero A, Novotni D, et al. Closed loop ventilation mode in intensive care unit: a randomized controlled clinical trial comparing the numbers of manual ventilator setting changes. Minerva Anestesiol 2018;84(1):58–67.
45. Dojat M, Harf A, Touchard D, et al. Evaluation of a knowledge-based system providing ventilatory management and decision for extubation. Am J Respir Crit Care Med 1996;153:997–1004.
46. Bouadma L, Lellouche F, Cabello B, et al. Computer-driven management of prolonged mechanical ventilation and weaning: a pilot study. Intensive Care Med 2005;31:1446–50.
47. Lellouche F, Mancebo J, Jolliet P, et al. A multicenter randomized trial of computer-driven protocolized weaning from mechanical ventilation. Am J Respir Crit Care Med 2006;174(8):894–900.
48. Rose L, Presneill JJ, Johnston L, et al. A randomised, controlled trial of conventional versus automated weaning from mechanical ventilation using SmartCare/PS. Intensive Care Med 2008;34:1788–95.
49. Jouvet P, Farges C, Hatzakis G, et al. Weaning children from mechanical ventilation with a computer-driven system (closed-loop protocol): a pilot study. Pediatr Crit Care Med 2007;8:425–32.
50. Kataoka G, Murai N, Kodera K, et al. Clinical experience with smart care after off-pump coronary artery bypass for early extubation. J Artif Organs 2007;10:218–22.
51. Schadler D, Engel C, Elke G, et al. Automatic control of pressure support for ventilator weaning in surgical intensive care patients. Am J Respir Crit Care Med 2012;185:637–44.
52. MacIntyre NR. Evidence-based guidelines for weaning and discontinuing ventilatory support. Chest 2001;120:375S–95S.
53. Burns KE, Lellouche F, Nisenbaum R, et al. Automated weaning and SBT systems versus non-automated weaning strategies for weaning time in invasively ventilated critically ill adults. Cochrane Database Syst Rev 2014;(9):CD008638.
54. Wenstedt EFE, De Bie Dekker AJR, Roos AN, et al. Current practice of closed-loop mechanical ventilation modes on intensive care units - a nationwide survey in the Netherlands. Neth J Med 2017;75:145–50.

Noninvasive Options

Giuseppe Bello, MD*, Alessandra Ionescu Maddalena, MD,
Valentina Giammatteo, MD, Massimo Antonelli, MD

KEYWORDS

- Noninvasive ventilation • Critical care • Chronic obstructive pulmonary disease
- Pulmonary edema • Ventilator weaning • Equipment and supplies

KEY POINTS

- Noninvasive ventilation should be considered in the management of critically ill patients with acute respiratory failure of various origins, particularly those with chronic obstructive pulmonary disease exacerbation and acute cardiogenic pulmonary edema.
- Noninvasive ventilation may have a role in preventing postextubation acute respiratory failure.
- Identifying patients who are proper candidates for noninvasive ventilation can help avoid inappropriate application of noninvasive ventilation or dangerous delays before endotracheal intubation.
- Patients at high risk of noninvasive ventilation failure should be managed only by experienced personnel, using an extremely prudent approach.
- The presence of strong inspiratory effort during noninvasive ventilation may result in non-protective ventilation, with excessive levels of transpulmonary pressure and a hidden lung overstretch even if airway pressures are not high.

INTRODUCTION

Noninvasive ventilation (NIV) refers to the provision of ventilatory assistance using techniques that do not bypass the upper airway. The main advantages of NIV over invasive ventilation include preventing complications related to endotracheal intubation (ETI), reducing patient discomfort, and maintaining airway protective mechanisms. NIV is now the recommended first-line method of ventilator support in selected patients with chronic obstructive pulmonary disease (COPD) exacerbation or acute cardiogenic pulmonary edema (CPE), and it has also been found useful to prevent postextubation acute respiratory failure (ARF).[1] The potential of avoiding complications of ETI, lowering morbidity and mortality rates in selected patients with ARF,

The authors declare that they have no commercial or financial conflicts of interest and no funding sources.
Department of Anesthesia and Intensive Care, Fondazione Policlinico Universitario Agostino Gemelli, Università Cattolica del Sacro Cuore, Largo A. Gemelli 8, Rome 00168, Italy
* Corresponding author.
E-mail address: gsppbll@gmail.com

Crit Care Clin 34 (2018) 395–412
https://doi.org/10.1016/j.ccc.2018.03.007
0749-0704/18/© 2018 Elsevier Inc. All rights reserved.

criticalcare.theclinics.com

has been the major driving force of the increasing use of NIV in the acute care setting over the past decades.

Currently, the utilization rates for NIV vary enormously among different acute care hospitals, mainly due to differences in physician knowledge, respiratory therapist training, and equipment availability. A French study in a large cohort of patients admitted to the ICU with ARF and the need of mechanical ventilation over a 15-year period (between 1997 and 2011) showed that the use of NIV increased steadily throughout the study period, up to 42% in 2011, and first-line NIV was associated with better 60-day survival and fewer ICU-acquired infections compared with first-line intubation.[2]

This article discusses the use of NIV in patients with ARF or who are at risk of ARF, focusing on the criteria for patient selection, choice of the interface, ventilator settings, and monitoring.

NONINVASIVE VENTILATION AND CONTINUOUS POSITIVE AIRWAY PRESSURE

The terms, *continuous positive airway pressure (CPAP)* and *NIV*, should not be used interchangeably. CPAP delivers a constant pressure throughout spontaneous inspiration and exhalation without assisting inspiration. Because spontaneous breathing is not assisted, this technique requires an intact respiratory drive and ability to accomplish adequate alveolar ventilation. CPAP increases functional residual capacity and opens underventilated alveoli, thus decreasing right-to-left intrapulmonary shunt and improving oxygenation and lung mechanics.[3] Moreover, CPAP may reduce the work of breathing and dyspnea in COPD patients by counterbalancing the inspiratory threshold load imposed by autointrinsic positive end-expiratory pressure (PEEP).[4] Finally, by lowering left ventricular transmural pressure in patients with left congestive heart failure, CPAP may reduce left ventricular afterload without compromising cardiac index.[5]

In contrast, NIV provides a pressure during the inspiratory phase greater than the pressure applied during exhalation, thus providing ventilatory support to unload respiratory muscles (**Fig. 1**). In hypoxemic patients, NIV has been demonstrated to improve dyspnea and gas exchange, lowering neuromuscular drive and inspiratory muscle effort, whereas CPAP used alone can improve oxygenation, but it is less effective in unloading respiratory muscles.[6]

NONINVASIVE VENTILATION AND HIGH-FLOW NASAL CANNULA OXYGENATION

High-flow nasal cannula oxygenation (HFNCO) (**Fig. 2**) is increasingly used in critically ill patients. Use of nasal prongs to deliver high heated and humidified flows (maximum 60 L/min) at a prescribed fraction of inspired oxygen (Fio_2) is an attractive alternative to conventional oxygen therapy. The main potential mechanisms through which HFNCO may alleviate symptoms of respiratory distress and enhance gas exchange include dead space washout with subsequent facilitation of carbon dioxide (CO_2) removal, provision of a moderate flow-dependent positive airway pressure, reduction in inspiratory nasopharyngeal resistance, and a better tolerance and comfort with the technique.[7] Levels of airway pressure (generally <4 cm H_2O) measured in the nasopharynx or the trachea increase as flow increases and are higher during breathing with mouth closed compared with mouth open.[8,9] **Table 1** describes the technical and physiologic aspects of noninvasive ventilation compared with HFNCO. Over the past years, some studies have compared HFNCO with NIV in the ICU, supporting the use of HFNCO in hypoxemic ARF patients having adequate muscular endurance[10]

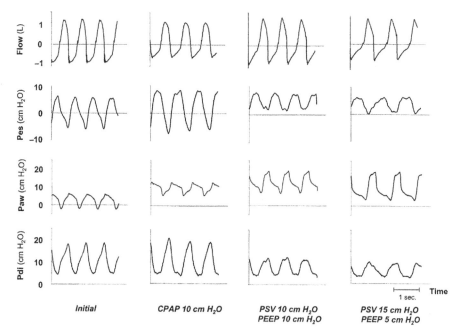

Fig. 1. Tracings of flow, esophageal pressure (Pes), airway pressure (Paw), and transdiaphragmatic pressure (Pdi) in a patient under spontaneous breathing, CPAP, and PSV. Compared with spontaneous breathing and CPAP, PSV periods were associated with decreased Pes and Pdi swings. (*From* L'Her E, Deye N, Lellouche F, et al. Physiologic effects of noninvasive ventilation during acute lung injury. Am J RespirCrit Care Med 2005;172:1112–8; with permission.)

or cardiothoracic surgical patients.[11] Further studies are needed, however, to define the actual role of HFNCO in the critical care setting.

INTERFACES OF NONINVASIVE VENTILATION

Interfaces connect ventilator tubing to the face of a patient, allowing the delivery of pressurized gas into the airway. Selection of a proper interface is a critical issue for the success of NIV.

Nasal Mask

The standard nasal mask (**Fig. 3**) is a triangular or cone-shaped clear plastic device that fits over the nose by a soft cushion or flange. Because of the pressure exerted over the bridge of the nose, the mask may cause skin irritation and redness, and even ulceration. Several types of strap systems have been used to hold the mask in place. Depending on the interface, straps attach at 2 or as many as 5 points on the mask and may be provided with hook-and-loop fasteners. A seal connector in the dome of the mask may be used for the passage of a nasogastric tube. Nasal masks are generally preferred in patients who need chronic administration of NIV.

Oronasal Mask

Oronasal or face masks cover both the nose and the mouth (**Fig. 4**). The oronasal mask is largely used in patients with copious air leaking through the mouth during

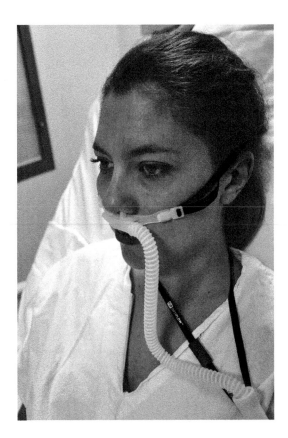

Fig. 2. HFNCO.

nasal mask ventilation. Interference with speech, eating, and expectoration and the likelihood of claustrophobic reactions are greater with oronasal than with nasal masks. In the acute setting, however, oronasal masks are preferable to nasal masks because dyspneic patients are mouth breathers, predisposing to greater air leakage during nasal mask ventilation. The oronasal masks, like the nasal mask, may cause facial skin breakdown, especially over the nasal bridge. As with the nasal mask, the positioning of a nasogastric tube (**Fig. 5**) may protect from gastric distension, even though this is not a common event.

A unique type of oronasal mask is the full-face mask (**Fig. 6**) which is made of clear plastic and uses a soft silicone flange that seals around the perimeter of the face, thereby avoiding direct pressure on facial structures. Over past years, new face mask models have been developed with the aim of improving patient comfort and interface performance. Characteristics of recent models of full-face mask include a lightweight design, a seal connector specifically dedicated to the passage of the feeding tube, a soft and thin membrane of the mask contour, and a mask holder that incorporates more than 4 points of attachment to secure the head straps.

Helmet

The standard helmet (**Fig. 7**) is a transparent hood that covers the entire head of the patient with a soft collar neck seal. The increase of pressure during ventilation makes the soft collar sealing comfortable to the neck and shoulders, avoiding air leakage. The

Table 1
Technical and physiologic aspects of noninvasive ventilation compared with high-flow nasal cannula oxygenation

	High-Flow Nasal Cannula Oxygenation	Noninvasive Ventilation
Ability to apply a predefined and constant level of PEEP	No	Yes
Ability to apply positive pressure during the inspiratory phase	No	Yes
Additional dead space	No	Yes (depending on the interface or the use of HME)
Problems of asynchrony	No	Yes (depending on the interface or ventilation mode)
Risk for skin breakdown	No	Yes (depending on the interface)
Compromised ability to speak or eat	No	Yes (depending on the interface)
Need of mechanical ventilator	No	Yes
Availability of respiratory monitoring (eg, tidal volume and minute ventilation) or respiratory alarms	No	Yes

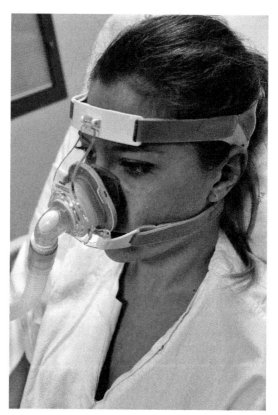

Fig. 3. Nasal mask.

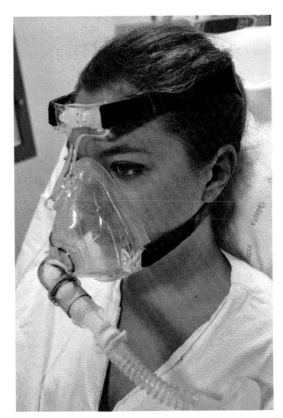

Fig. 4. Oronasal mask.

whole apparatus is connected to a mechanical ventilator by a standard respiratory circuit. The 2 ports of the helmet act as inlet and outlet for inspiratory and expiratory gas flows, and a specific connector placed in the plastic ring can be used to allow the passage of a nasogastric tube. In some versions, a security valve is located on the helmet to reduce the risk of asphyxia. The patient is allowed to drink through a straw or to be fed a liquid diet. The main advantages of the helmet include good tolerability, with a satisfactory interaction of the patient with the environment; lower risk of dermal lesions; and, compared with the mask, easier applicability to any patient regardless of the face contour. In a recent model of helmet, a zip opening ensures patient accessibility without the need to remove the interface, and alternative fastening systems on the top of the helmet can avoid skin damage along the armpit braces.

CARBON DIOXIDE REBREATHING DURING NONINVASIVE VENTILATION

NIV interfaces behave differently in respect to CO_2 exchange. The face mask constitutes an additional mechanical dead space, and its effect on CO_2 rebreathing is proportional to its internal volume.[12] Because this volume is small compared with a patient's tidal volume, the amount of CO_2 that is rebreathed is also small. In contrast, CO_2 exchange during helmet ventilation follows the model of a semiclosed environment, such as a closed room provided with an air exchange system.[13] According to this model, the factors determining CO_2 concentration inside the helmet are the

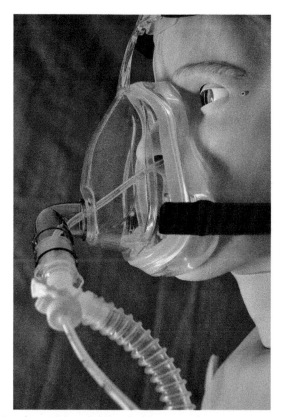

Fig. 5. Nasogastric tube positioned through the oronasal mask.

amount of CO_2 produced by the patient and the fresh gas flow that flushes the helmet. As a result, the volume of the helmet has no direct effect on the CO_2 concentration but only on the rate at which a given CO_2 concentration is reached.

When CPAP is delivered by the helmet, the inspired P_{CO_2} seems independent of the level of CPAP and inversely correlated to the fresh gas flow delivered.[14] High gas flows of 45 L/min to 60 L/min render the CO_2 rebreathing clinically irrelevant during helmet CPAP.[14] Compared with CPAP, helmet-delivered NIV in pressure support ventilation (PSV) mode can provide a more efficient CO_2 washout, probably because of the phasic administration of inspiratory flow during such a ventilatory mode.[15] In addition, the analysis of CO_2 rebreathing during helmet-delivered PSV does not show any significant reduction in inspired CO_2 after increasing the level of inspiratory assistance.[15] Using a sophisticated computational fluid dynamic model to evaluate the effective dead space between different NIV interfaces, Fodil and colleagues[16] showed that the dead space differed only modestly (110–370 mL) between the face mask and the helmet, whereas their internal volumes were markedly different (110–10,000 mL). Such data confirm that effective dead space is not related to the internal gas volume included inside the interface.

ASYNCHRONY DURING NONINVASIVE VENTILATION

Synchrony between a patient's spontaneous breathing and the ventilator set parameters is one of the key factors affecting tolerance to NIV. The lack of an optimal

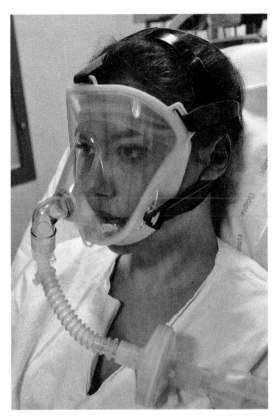

Fig. 6. Full-face mask.

patient-ventilator interaction can result in increased work of breathing and patient discomfort.[17] Patient-ventilator asynchrony is recognized as events that include ineffective triggering, double-triggering, autotriggering, premature cycling, and delayed cycling.

When PSV is used as a noninvasive ventilatory assistance mode, some forms of patient-ventilator asynchrony may occur, causing breathing discomfort. In a prospective multicenter observation study on ARF patients receiving NIV via a face mask in PSV mode, the level of pressure support and the magnitude of leaks were significantly associated with asynchrony.[18] Eventual air leaks during noninvasive PSV may impede the adequate reduction in inspiratory flow required to open the expiratory valve, thus prolonging the inspiratory flow. In these circumstances, air leaks can be minimized by optimizing the fitting or size of the interface or even switching to another type of interface. To reduce leaks, it may also be helpful to decrease ventilator pressure settings as much as allowed by ventilatory parameters. When air leaking occurs, an option to obtain a better patient-machine interaction is to select pressure-limited, time-cycled ventilation modes, or even PSV mode with a set maximal inspiratory time, when offered by the machine used. Additionally, with ventilators that allow changing the expiratory trigger, raising the cycling off airflow threshold (ie, the percentage of peak inspiratory flow at which transition from inspiration to expiration occurs) can activate an earlier switchover to expiration, thus avoiding prolonged insufflations and patient-ventilator asynchrony.

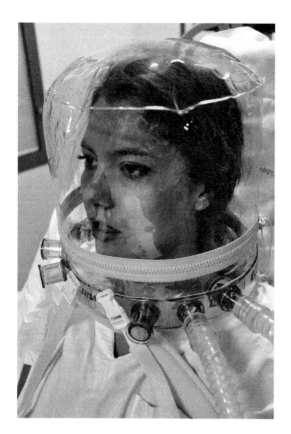

Fig. 7. Helmet.

In new ventilators, an NIV mode algorithm measures and compensates for leaks to minimize their detrimental impact on patient-ventilator synchrony. In the presence of significant air leaks, pressure-targeted modes are preferred to deliver NIV because they can maintain delivered tidal volume better than volume-targeted modes.[19]

During helmet-delivered NIV, the pressure delivered by the ventilator is partially spent to pressurize the large inner volume of the helmet, with a lower level of assistance in the initial phase of the breathing effort. Additionally, given the mechanical characteristics of the helmet, expiratory trigger efficiency also might be adversely affected, thus worsening patient-ventilator asynchrony. Accordingly, increasing both PEEP and pressure support level and using the highest pressurization rate are advisable when NIV is applied with the helmet, to increase the effective elastance of the system and enhance the trigger sensitivity.[20]

MAIN INDICATIONS FOR NONINVASIVE VENTILATION

Over the past 2 decades, NIV has come to assume a pivotal role in the supportive therapy for ARF requiring ICU admission, particularly for some clinical conditions that include COPD exacerbations, CPE, immunocompromise, and ventilator weaning.

Chronic Obstructive Pulmonary Disease Exacerbation

In patients with ARF due to acute exacerbations of COPD, the use of NIV has proved effective in ameliorating dyspnea, improving vital signs and gas exchange, preventing

ETI, and improving hospital survival.[1] There is now general agreement concerning the early use of NIV in such patients. In a large 10-year (from 1998 to 2008) prevalence study of more than 7 million patients with acute COPD exacerbations, a 462% increase in NIV use and a 42% decline in invasive mechanical ventilation use were observed.[21]

In COPD patients with acute respiratory decompensation, the increased flow resistance and the impossibility to complete expiration before inspiration determine high levels of dynamic hyperinflation and substantial shortening of the diaphragm and accessory respiratory muscles, thus reducing mechanical efficiency and endurance. The need to overcome inspiratory threshold load due to auto-PEEP and to drive tidal volume against airway resistances increases the respiratory muscle fatigue. With NIV, the combination of external PEEP and PSV offsets the auto-PEEP level and reduces the work of breathing.[22]

At present, NIV should be considered the first-line therapeutic option to prevent ETI and improve outcome in patients with exacerbations of COPD who have no contraindication to NIV.

Cardiogenic Pulmonary Edema

Noninvasive use of positive airway pressure should be strongly considered as a first-line treatment in patients with CPE. Both NIV and CPAP have proved to efficiently improve respiratory distress during CPE.[1] Because both CPAP and bilevel NIV have showed similar efficacy in decreasing the need for ETI and mortality without increasing the risk of acute myocardial infarction, CPAP could be considered the preferred intervention in CPE patients, because it is cheaper and easier to use in various clinical settings.

Immunocompromise

NIV plays a central role in the management of immunocompromised patients, because respiratory failure is the main indication for ICU admission in these patients. Currently available literature is, for the most part, supportive of the use of NIV as the first-line approach for treating mild/moderate ARF in selected patients with immunosuppression of various origins. Although most of the studies have proved clinical benefits of NIV or CPAP in immunocompromised patients,[23–27] in a more recent multicenter RCT, however, some investigators could not confirm the benefits of NIV over standard oxygen therapy in these patients.[28]

Weaning

NIV use has been proposed as prophylaxis to prevent reintubation (preventive NIV) or as rescue intervention in case of established postextubation respiratory failure (rescue NIV). Importantly, in patients with specific risk factors for ARF after extubation, application of NIV immediately after extubation was efficiently used as a tool to prevent postextubation ARF.[29,30] No benefits were found, however, in avoiding reintubation in patients who had already developed ARF after extubation, because they showed higher mortality rates compared with patients treated according to standard treatment.[31,32] Hence, even though NIV approach can be helpful in preventing postextubation ARF, more data are needed to better define which patient categories may most benefit from its use in such field.

OTHER APPLICATIONS OF NONINVASIVE VENTILATION
De Novo Acute Respiratory Failure

De novo ARF is defined as a respiratory failure not exacerbating a preexisting respiratory disease (COPD or restrictive, such as obesity hypoventilation syndrome or neuromuscular disease) or cardiac insufficiency. It is also called hypoxemic ARF. Patients with hypoxemic ARF are also defined as those with a ratio of Pao_2 to Fio_2 of 300 mm Hg or less, acute dyspnea (with a respiratory rate >25 breaths/min and/or active contraction of accessory respiratory muscles) and $Paco_2$ below or equal to 45 mm Hg. In contrast to COPD, the efficacy of NIV in patients with de novo ARF is less clear. The pathophysiologic mechanisms that underlie hypoxemia include shunt, ventilation/ perfusion abnormalities, and impairment of alveolar-capillary diffusion.

In acute respiratory distress syndrome (ARDS),[33] transient loss of positive pressure during mechanical ventilation may seriously compromise lung recruitment and gas exchange. For this reason, most NIV studies have excluded patients with ARDS, and few data are currently available on this topic. A subset analysis of 2 RCTs showed that in patients with ARDS (n = 31), NIV avoided ETI in 60% of the cases.[24,34]

A study of NIV use in French and Belgian ICUs over a 15-year period (between 1997 and 2011) showed an increase in the overall use of NIV over time and a reduction in NIV use in patients with de novo ARF.[35] In these patients, NIV failure was no longer associated with mortality as in previous years, suggesting a better selection of patients for NIV therapy and greater expertise of caregivers in the application and termination of NIV during recent years.

In view of this, NIV can be used to treat patients with de novo ARF, as long as an extremely prudent approach is adopted, limiting the application of NIV to hemodynamically stable patients who can be closely monitored in the ICU, where ETI is promptly available. Patients at high risk of failure should be closely managed and only by experienced personnel maintaining a low threshold for ETI.

Postoperative

CPAP or NIV application may be considered a suitable option for the management of patients after thoracic and upper abdominal surgery who frequently develop prolonged postoperative gas exchange deterioration and reduction in functional residual capacity. A systematic review summarized the results of 29 articles where the use of preventive and therapeutic NIV was investigated in postsurgical patients after thoracoabdominal/bariatric surgical interventions and solid organ transplants.[36] Arterial blood gas improvement and intubation rate reduction were the main benefits associated with the use of NIV. A more recent multicenter randomized controlled trial (RCT) on postoperative patients after abdominal surgery confirmed the benefits of NIV in this setting.[37] Thus, accumulating evidence supports the use of NIV/CPAP in reducing respiratory postoperative complications in selected patients.

Trauma

Posttraumatic acute respiratory failure usually results from reduced pulmonary compliance and functional residual capacity and subsequent restrictive defects. In a meta-analysis of 10 studies addressing the use of NIV in patients with chest trauma associated with mild to severe respiratory failure, there was no difference between CPAP and pressure support NIV in terms of mortality, but the latter significantly increased arterial oxygenation, leading to a reduction in intubation rate and infectious complications incidence.[38] Despite the favorable results obtained, however, large randomized studies are still needed before definitive recommendations on the use of NIV in posttraumatic ARF can be made.

End of Life

NIV may have a role in the management of terminal patients with respiratory failure. In these patients, caregivers should remember that not assuring a quality death to the patient is a serious and irreparable error. Use of NIV in patients with a do-not-resuscitate order still remains a matter of concern, with some warning of the potential ethical and economic cost of delaying the inevitable in patients with terminal respiratory failure.[39,40] In end-of-life patients with ARF, NIV may be of benefit because it may alleviate dyspnea and prolong life for a period of time sufficient to possibly carry out personal tasks or realize end-of-life desires. Prior to initiation of NIV in terminally ill patients, family members and clinicians should have a clear understanding of the possible outcomes of NIV.

PRACTICAL ADVICE

Fig. 8 shows the sequential steps for applying NIV in patients with ARF.

Patient Selection

NIV should be considered early when patients develop signs of incipient respiratory failure, such as dyspnea, tachypnea, accessory muscle use, paradoxic abdominal breathing, and gas exchange deterioration.

NIV should be avoided in the following conditions:

1. Coma, seizures, or severe central neurologic disturbances
2. Inability to protect the airway or clear respiratory secretions
3. Unstable hemodynamic conditions (blood pressure or rhythm instability)
4. Upper airway obstruction
5. Severe upper gastrointestinal bleeding
6. Recent facial surgery, trauma, burns, deformity, or inability to fit the interface
7. Recent gastroesophageal surgery
8. Undrained pneumothorax
9. Recurrent vomiting

Even though patients with altered levels of consciousness due to hypercapnic ARF are exposed to high risk of NIV failure, a cautious attempt with NIV may be performed

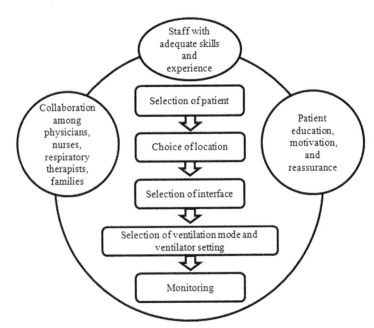

Fig. 8. Practical advice for the application of NIV in patients with acute respiratory failure.

in those lethargic hypercapnic patients who otherwise are good candidates for NIV, provided that careful monitoring is available and prompt ETI is accessible.[41]

Predictors of Noninvasive Ventilation Success or Failure

Identification of predictors of success or failure may help in recognizing patients who are likely to benefit from NIV and exclude those for whom NIV would be unsafe or ineffective, avoiding dangerous delays before ETI. Moreover, knowing these factors may be useful in deciding the duration of the trial of NIV.

Box 1[42–47] summarizes predictors of NIV failure observed in COPD and hypoxemic patients.

Selection of Ventilation Modes

Each ventilation mode has theoretic advantages and limitations. Choosing the right ventilation mode is crucial for achieving physiologic and clinical benefit during NIV.

Spontaneously breathing patients with respiratory failure of various etiologies may benefit from CPAP to correct hypoxemia. A growing body of evidence supports the use of CPAP or NIV as a first-line intervention in patients with CPE.[1] As in the intubated mechanically ventilated patients, application of external PEEP counterbalances the effects of dynamic hyperinflation in patients with acute exacerbation of COPD. In these patients, NIV performed by different ventilator modes can provide respiratory muscle

---

Box 1
Predictors of failure of noninvasive ventilation

COPD patients

- Lower arterial pH at baseline[42,43]
- Greater severity of illness, as indicated by APACHE II score[44]
- Inability to coordinate with the ventilator[44]
- Inability to minimize the amount of mouth leak with nasal mask ventilation[44]
- Less efficient or less rapid correction of hypercapnia, pH, or tachypnea in the early hours[44]
- Functional limitations caused by COPD before ICU admission, evaluated using a score correlated to home activities of daily living[43]
- Higher number of medical complications (in particular, hyperglycemia) on ICU admission[43]

Hypoxemic patients

- Higher severity score (SAPS II ≥ 35[45]/SAPS II >34[46]/higher SAPS II[24])
- Older age (>40 years)[45]
- Presence of ARDS or community-acquired pneumonia[24,27,45]
- Failure to improve oxygenation after 1 hour of treatment (Pao_2:Fio_2 ≤ 146 mm Hg[45]/Pao_2:Fio_2 ≤ 175 mm Hg[46])
- Higher respiratory rate under NIV[27]
- Need for vasopressors[27]
- Need for renal replacement therapy[27]
- Expired tidal volume above 9.5 mL/kg PBW in patients with Pao_2:Fio_2 ≤ 200 mm Hg[47]

Abbreviations: APACHE, Acute Physiology and Chronic Health Evaluation; SAPS, Simplified Acute Physiology Score.

rest and improve respiratory physiologic parameters.[48] Volume-controlled ventilation mode can be useful in patients with severe chest wall deformity or obesity who may need higher inflation pressures.

Triggering systems are critical to the success of NIV in both assist and control modes. During assisted ventilation, flow triggering reduces breathing effort more effectively compared with pressure triggering, obtaining a better patient-ventilator interaction.[49]

In the absence of evidence favoring a specific ventilatory mode, the choice of ventilation mode should be dictated by factors, such as personal experience, operation setting, etiology, and severity of the pathologic process responsible for ARF. Assisted modes, however, in particular PSV, are usually best tolerated and can be safely and effectively performed.

Setting the Ventilator

For pressure-targeted ventilation, it is suggested to start at low pressures to facilitate patient tolerance (appropriate initial pressures are a CPAP of 3 cm H_2O–5 cm H_2O and an inspiratory pressure of 8 cm H_2O–12 cm H_2O above CPAP) and, if necessary, gradually increase pressure settings as tolerated to alleviate dyspnea, decrease respiratory rate, achieve adequate exhaled tidal volume (between 6 mL/kg predicted body weight [PBW] and 8 mL/kg PBW), and establish good patient-ventilator interaction. Pressures commonly used to administer CPAP in patients with ARF range from 5 cm H_2O to 12 cm H_2O. Oxygen supplementation should be provided as needed to keep oxygen saturation above 92% or between 85% and 90% in patients at risk of worsening hypercapnia. A modality that provides a backup rate is needed for patients with inadequate or unstable ventilatory drive.

Sedation

Although sedation is infrequently required during NIV, caution is advised if benzodiazepines or opiates are administered to prevent hypoventilation or loss of airway protection. During recent years, dexmedetomidine has been increasingly used in the clinical practice as a sedative agent, although few data are available in patients undergoing NIV.[50]

Monitoring

Monitoring of patients receiving NIV has the aim to determine whether NIV is performed safely and effectively. Monitoring of patients under NIV in the acute care setting includes

1. Level of consciousness
2. Comfort
3. Chest wall motion
4. Accessory muscle recruitment
5. Patient-ventilator synchrony
6. Respiratory rate
7. Exhaled tidal volume
8. Flow and pressure waveforms
9. Heart rate
10. Blood pressure
11. Continuous electrocardiography
12. Continuous oximetry
13. Arterial blood gas at baseline, after 1 hour to 2 hours, and as clinically indicated.

ETI must be rapidly initiated, when indicated. Criteria used to perform ETI in ARF patients undergoing NIV are as follows:

1. Patient intolerance
2. Inability to improve gas exchange
3. Inability to improve dyspnea or respiratory muscle fatigue
4. Appearance of severe hemodynamic or electrocardiographic instability
5. Severe neurologic deterioration

Humidification During Noninvasive Ventilation

Despite encouraging early results on the physiologic benefits of heated humidifiers (HHs) in minimizing work of breathing and improving CO_2 clearance compared with heat and moisture exchangers (HMEs) in patients receiving NIV, a multicenter RCT on the use of HH or HME in hypoxemic or hypercapnic NIV patients found no differences between the HH group and HME group in terms of NIV duration, ICU and hospital length of stay, or ICU mortality.[51]

INTENSITY OF INSPIRATORY EFFORTS AND LUNG STRETCHING DURING NONINVASIVE VENTILATION

When spontaneous breathing is preserved during mechanical ventilation, as in the case of NIV, caregivers should be aware that the presence of strong inspiratory effort can result in a nonprotective ventilation, with excessive levels of transpulmonary pressure and a hidden lung overstretch, even if applied airway pressures are not high.

On the other hand, compared with fully controlled mechanical ventilation, gentle spontaneous breathing during ventilatory assistance offers several potential benefits, but vigorous efforts can be detrimental for lung tissue and clinical outcomes. Tidal volume is of relevant importance during assisted spontaneous breathing. In a multicenter study on the association between expired tidal volume and NIV outcome in 62 patients with hypoxemic ARF, Carteaux and colleagues[47] found that a higher expired tidal volume was independently associated with NIV failure. In particular, an expired tidal volume above 9.5 mL/kg PBW could accurately predict NIV failure when patients had a Pao_2:Fio_2 ratio less than or equal to 200 mm Hg, suggesting that persistently high tidal volumes were mainly driven by continued strong patient inspiratory efforts. In 10 patients undergoing different levels of PSV followed by a phase of controlled mechanical ventilation, Bellani and colleagues[52] compared the amplitude of the change in transpulmonary pressure during spontaneous assisted breathing and fully controlled ventilation, trying to match similar conditions of airflow and volume. Under similar conditions of flow and volume, transpulmonary pressure change was similar between controlled mechanical ventilation and PSV. Furthermore, decreasing levels of pressure support assistance led to progressively more negative changes in transpulmonary pressure, causing remarkably negative swings also in alveolar pressure, a mechanism by which spontaneous breathing might potentially induce lung damage.

SUMMARY

To date, the best-established indication for NIV is ARF related to COPD exacerbations or CPE. Various categories of hypoxemic non-COPD patients, in particular those with immunosuppression or in the postoperative setting may also benefit from NIV, providing they are managed in centers with extensive experience in the use of NIV. Interfaces are continually improving, and NIV is increasingly proposed to assist ventilator weaning process in selected patients under invasive mechanical ventilation. Effective and safe use of NIV requires awareness of its potential for harm as well as benefit. Further studies may be useful in clarifying the actual role of HFNCO, compared with NIV, in the management of acute respiratory failure.

REFERENCES

1. Rochwerg B, Brochard L, Elliott MW, et al. Official ERS/ATS clinical practice guidelines: noninvasive ventilation for acute respiratory failure. Eur Respir J 2017;50:1602426.

2. Schnell D, Timsit JF, Darmon M, et al. Noninvasive mechanical ventilation in acute respiratory failure: trends in use and outcomes. Intensive Care Med 2014;40:582–91.

3. Katz JA, Marks JD. Inspiratory work with and without continuous positive airway pressure in patients with acute respiratory failure. Anesthesiology 1985;63:598–607.

4. Petrof BJ, Legaré M, Goldberg P, et al. Continuous positive airway pressure reduces work of breathing and dyspnea during weaning from mechanical ventilation in severe chronic obstructive pulmonary disease. Am Rev Respir Dis 1990;141:281–9.

5. Naughton MT, Rahman MA, Hara K, et al. Effect of continuous positive airway pressure on intrathoracic and left ventricular transmural pressures in patients with congestive heart failure. Circulation 1995;91:1725–31.

6. L'Her E, Deye N, Lellouche F, et al. Physiologic effects of noninvasive ventilation during acute lung injury. Am J Respir Crit Care Med 2005;172:1112–8.

7. Papazian L, Corley A, Hess D, et al. Use of high-flow nasal cannula oxygenation in ICU adults: a narrative review. Intensive Care Med 2016;42:1336–49.

8. Parke RL, McGuinness SP. Pressures delivered by nasal high flow oxygen during all phases of the respiratory cycle. Respir Care 2013;58:1621–4.

9. Chanques G, Riboulet F, Molinari N, et al. Comparison of three high flow oxygen therapy delivery devices: a clinical physiological cross-over study. Minerva Anestesiol 2013;79:1344–55.

10. Frat JP, Thille AW, Mercat A, et al, FLORALI Study Group, REVA Network. High-flow oxygen through nasal cannula in acute hypoxemic respiratory failure. N Engl J Med 2015;372:2185–96.

11. Stéphan F, Barrucand B, Petit P, et al, BiPOP Study Group. High-flow nasal oxygen vs noninvasive positive airway pressure in hypoxemic patients after cardiothoracic surgery: a randomized clinical trial. JAMA 2015;13:2331–9.

12. Criner GJ, Travaline JM, Brennan KJ, et al. Efficacy of a new full face mask for noninvasive positive pressure ventilation. Chest 1994;106:1109–15.

13. Taccone P, Hess D, Caironi P, et al. Continuous positive airway pressure delivered with a "helmet": effects on carbon dioxide rebreathing. Crit Care Med 2004;32:2090–6.

14. Patroniti N, Foti G, Manfio A, et al. Head helmet versus face mask for non-invasive continuous positive airway pressure: a physiological study. Intensive Care Med 2003;29:1680–7.

15. Costa R, Navalesi P, Antonelli M, et al. Physiologic evaluation of different levels of assistance during noninvasive ventilation delivered through a helmet. Chest 2005;128:2984–90.

16. Fodil R, Lellouche F, Mancebo J, et al. Comparison of patient–ventilator interfaces based on their computerized effective dead space. Intensive Care Med 2011;37:257–62.

17. Kondili E, Prinianakis G, Georgopoulos D. Patient-ventilator interaction. Br J Anaesth 2003;91:106–19.

18. Vignaux L, Vargas F, Roeseler J, et al. Patient-ventilator asynchrony during non-invasive ventilation for acute respiratory failure: a multicenter study. Intensive Care Med 2009;35:840–6.
19. Mehta S, McCool FD, Hill NS. Leak compensation in positive pressure ventilators: a lung model study. Eur Respir J 2001;17:259–67.
20. Vargas F, Thille A, Lyazidi A, et al. Helmet with specific settings versus facemask for noninvasive ventilation. Crit Care Med 2009;37:1921–8.
21. Chandra D, Stamm JA, Taylor B, et al. Outcomes of noninvasive ventilation for acute exacerbations of chronic obstructive pulmonary disease in the United States, 1998-2008. Am J Respir Crit Care Med 2012;185:152–9.
22. Appendini L, Purro A, Patessio A, et al. Partitioning of inspiratory muscle work-load and pressure assistance in ventilator-dependent COPD patients. Am J Respir Crit Care Med 1996;154:1301–9.
23. Gristina GR, Antonelli M, Conti G, et al. Noninvasive versus invasive ventilation for acute respiratory failure in patients with hematologic malignancies: a 5-year multicenter observational survey. Crit Care Med 2011;39:2232–9.
24. Antonelli M, Conti C, Bufi M, et al. Noninvasive ventilation for treatment of acute respiratory failure in patients undergoing solid organ transplantation. JAMA 2000; 283:235–41.
25. Hilbert G, Gruson D, Vargas F, et al. Noninvasive ventilation in immunosuppressed patients with pulmonary infiltrates, fever, and acute respiratory failure. N Engl J Med 2001;344:481–7.
26. Squadrone V, Massaia M, Bruno B, et al. Early CPAP prevents evolution of acute lung injury in patients with hematologic malignancy. Intensive Care Med 2010;36: 1666–74.
27. Adda M, Coquet I, Darmon M, et al. Predictors of noninvasive ventilation failure in patients with hematologic malignancy and acute respiratory failure. Crit Care Med 2008;36:2766–72.
28. Lemiale V, Mokart D, Resche-Rigon M, et al. Groupe de recherche en réanimation respiratoire du patient d'onco-hématologie (GRRR-OH). Effect of noninvasive ventilation vs oxygen therapy on mortality among immunocompromised patients with acute respiratory failure: a randomized clinical trial. JAMA 2015;314:1711–9.
29. Nava S, Gregoretti C, Fanfulla F, et al. Noninvasive ventilation to prevent respiratory failure after extubation in high-risk patients. Crit Care Med 2005;33:2465–70.
30. Ferrer M, Valencia M, Nicolas JM, et al. Early noninvasive ventilation averts extubation failure in patients at risk: a randomized trial. Am J Respir Crit Care Med 2006;173:164–70.
31. Keenan SP, Powers C, McCormack DG, et al. Noninvasive positive-pressure ventilation for postextubation respiratory distress: a randomized controlled trial. JAMA 2002;287:3238–44.
32. Esteban A, Frutos-Vivar F, Ferguson ND, et al. Noninvasive positive-pressure ventilation for respiratory failure after extubation. N Engl J Med 2004;350: 2452–60.
33. ARDS Definition Task Force, Ranieri VM, Rubenfeld GD, Thompson BT, et al. Acute respiratory distress syndrome: the Berlin definition. JAMA 2012;307: 2526–33.
34. Antonelli M, Conti G, Rocco M, et al. A comparison of noninvasive positive-pressure ventilation and conventional mechanical ventilation in patients with acute respiratory failure. N Engl J Med 1998;339:429–35.
35. Demoule A, Chevret S, Carlucci A, et al, oVNI Study Group, REVA Network (Research Network in Mechanical Ventilation). Changing use of noninvasive

ventilation in critically ill patients: trends over 15 years in francophone countries. Intensive Care Med 2016;42:82–92.

36. Chiumello D, Chevallard G, Gregoretti C. Non-invasive ventilation in postoperative patients: a systematic review. Intensive Care Med 2011;37:918–29.

37. Jaber S, Lescot T, Futier E, et al. Effect of noninvasive ventilation on tracheal reintubation among patients with hypoxemic respiratory failure following abdominal surgery: a randomized clinical trial. JAMA 2016;315:1345–53.

38. Chiumello D, Coppola S, Froio S, et al. Noninvasive ventilation in chest trauma: systematic review and meta-analysis. Intensive Care Med 2013;39:1171–80.

39. Clarke DE, Vaughan L, Raffin TA. Noninvasive positive pressure ventilation for patients with terminal respiratory failure: the ethical and economic costs of delaying the inevitable are too great. Am J Crit Care 1994;3:4–5.

40. Azoulay E, Kouatchet A, Jaber S, et al. Noninvasive mechanical ventilation in patients having declined tracheal intubation. Intensive Care Med 2013;39:292–301.

41. Díaz GG, Alcaraz AC, Talavera JC, et al. Noninvasive positive-pressure ventilation to treat hypercapnic coma secondary to respiratory failure. Chest 2005;127: 952–60.

42. Ambrosino N, Foglio K, Rubini F, et al. Non-invasive mechanical ventilation in acute respiratory failure due to chronic obstructive pulmonary disease: correlates for success. Thorax 1995;50:755–7.

43. Moretti M, Cilione C, Tampieri A, et al. Incidence and causes of non-invasive mechanical ventilation failure after initial success. Thorax 2000;55:819–25.

44. Soo Hoo GW, Santiago S, Williams AJ. Nasal mechanical ventilation for hypercapnic respiratory failure in chronic obstructive pulmonary disease: determinants of success and failure. Crit Care Med 1994;22:1253–61.

45. Antonelli M, Conti G, Moro ML, et al. Predictors of failure of noninvasive positive pressure ventilation in patients with acute hypoxemic respiratory failure: a multicenter study. Intensive Care Med 2001;27:1718–28.

46. Antonelli M, Conti G, Esquinas A, et al. A multiple-center survey on the use in clinical practice of noninvasive ventilation as a first-line intervention for acute respiratory distress syndrome. Crit Care Med 2007;35:18–25.

47. Carteaux G, Millán-Guilarte T, De Prost N, et al. Failure of noninvasive ventilation for de novo acute hypoxemic respiratory failure: role of tidal volume. Crit Care Med 2016;44:282–90.

48. Vitacca M, Rubini F, Foglio K, et al. Non-invasive modalities of positive pressure ventilation improve the outcome of acute exacerbations in COLD patients. Intensive Care Med 1993;19:450–5.

49. Nava S, Ambrosino N, Bruschi C, et al. Physiological effects of flow and pressure triggering during non invasive mechanical ventilation in patients with chronic obstructive pulmonary disease. Thorax 1997;52:249–54.

50. Huang Z, Chen YS, Yang ZL, et al. Dexmedetomidine versus midazolam for the sedation of patients with non-invasive ventilation failure. Intern Med 2012;51: 2299–305.

51. Lellouche F, L'Her E, Abroug F, et al. Impact of the humidification device on intubation rate during noninvasive ventilation with ICU ventilators: results of a multicenter randomized controlled trial. Intensive Care Med 2014;40:211–9.

52. Bellani G, Grasselli G, Teggia-Droghi M, et al. Do spontaneous and mechanical breathing have similar effects on average transpulmonary and alveolar pressure? A clinical crossover study. Crit Care 2016;20:142.

Extracorporeal Gas Exchange

Onnen Moerer, MD[a], Francesco Vasques, MD[b], Eleonora Duscio, MD[c], Francesco Cipulli, MD[d], Federica Romitti, MD[a], Luciano Gattinoni, MD[a], Michael Quintel, MD[a],*

KEYWORDS

- Critical care • Respiratory failure • Acute respiratory distress syndrome
- Mechanical ventilation • Extracorporeal gas exchange
- Extracorporeal membrane oxygenation (ECMO) • Extracorporeal CO_2 removal

KEY POINTS

- The transfer of O_2 and CO_2 via a selective membrane that separates gas and blood is a basic tenet of life.
- ECMO integrates an additional, "external" option for gas exchange into the circulation, the artificial lung mimics the principle of the native lungs.
- Extracorporeal gas exchange is a powerful tool. However, deeper understanding of the interactions between native and artificial lung, monitoring with better technologies, physiologic and observational studies and, patience are needed to avoid multicenter studies leading to results that carry a high risk to impede a successful further development.

INTRODUCTION

The transfer of O_2 and CO_2 via a selective membrane that separates gas and blood is a basic tenet of life. The lungs represent the first and last membrane to pass between the external environment and human body, allowing oxygen uptake and carbon dioxide delivery to happen. Any serious change in the integrity and functionality of the lungs potentially threatens life. Acute respiratory failure is characterized by hypoxemia, mostly caused by a marked increase of pulmonary shunt and impaired CO_2 removal caused by the inability of the respiratory muscles to move enough gas into heavy, edematous lungs to ensure a minute volume adequate to remove the CO_2 dissolved in plasma at an appropriate rate. These 2 impairments exist in parallel, but their degree of influence

a Department of Anesthesiology and Intensive Care Medicine, University Hospital, Georg-August University of Göttingen, Robert Koch Straße 40, Göttingen 37075, Germany; b Department of Medicine (DMED), Anesthesia and Intensive Care Unit, Padua University Hospital, Via C.Battisti, 267, Padua 35128, Italy; c Department of Pathophysiology and Transplantation, University of Milan, via F. Sforza 35, Milano 20122, Italy; d Dipartimento di Medicina e Chirurgia, Università degli Studi di Milano Bicocca, Piazza dell'Ateneo Nuovo 1, Milano 20126, Italy
* Corresponding author.
E-mail address: mquintel@med.uni-goettingen.de

Crit Care Clin 34 (2018) 413–422
https://doi.org/10.1016/j.ccc.2018.03.011
0749-0704/18/© 2018 Elsevier Inc. All rights reserved.

criticalcare.theclinics.com

might vary. In severe forms of acute respiratory failure like acute respiratory distress syndrome (ARDS), oxygenation and CO_2 removal represent equivalent treatment challenges, although only hypoxemia might cause an acutely life-threatening state. The classical and established treatment option is mechanical ventilation. However, mechanical ventilation has its own adverse effects, described as ventilator-induced lung injury (VILI), caused by the mechanical power transmitted to the lungs during ventilation and high fractions of inspired oxygen, leading either to direct destruction of the pulmonary matrix (barotrauma) or to the initiation or perpetuation of an inflammatory reaction of the lungs.[1] Another article in this issue deals with the causation of VILI and suggests an approach to its avoidance by conventional means.

Increasing knowledge about the negative adverse effects of mechanical ventilation and the technical development of artificial lungs mimicking the aveolo-capillary membrane while using silicone as membrane stimulated the conceptual idea to supportively use extracorporeal gas exchange during mechanical ventilation.[2] In the beginning, the objective to reduce the FiO_2 was the main driver for its use. Later on, the possibility to reduce the invasiveness of mechanical ventilation gained more importance when deciding about the use of extracorporeal gas exchange. In 1972, Hill and colleagues[3] reported the first successful treatment of an ARDS patient using a Bramson membrane lung for a period of 72 hours. In 1976, Bartlett[4] successfully treated the first newborn. Influenced by the oxygenator, the technique was reported as extracorporeal membrane oxygenation (ECMO). At that time, the ECMO technique, also used for respiratory support, was applied in the veno-arterial VA-mode.

In brief, an ECMO unit consists of a driving force, today mostly realized by a centrifugal pump, a gas exchanging unit, and mostly implemented as a hollow fiber membrane oxygenator, connecting tubing, and 2 single-stage or 1 double-stage cannula(s) for vascular drainage and return. The double stage cannula is by definition linked to veno-venous (VV)-ECMO, while single-stage cannulas are suitable for both the VA and VV modes. For respiratory support, the VV approach has become standard of care; in extreme cases, a hybrid solution combining VV with partial arterial return might be used.

In the ECMO unit, the oxygenator surface and blood flow are key determinants of oxygen transfer, whereas oxygenator surface and gas flow through the membrane lung (sweep gas) are key determinants of CO_2 removal. Consequently, if oxygenation is an issue, high blood flow rates are required; conversely, if decarboxylation is the goal, relatively low blood flow rates are needed to remove reasonable amounts of CO_2. The intended goals of extracorporeal support therefore largely influence the unit to choose (oxygenator size, cannula, and tubing size). Beside the artificial surface per se, the mechanical power created by the pump stresses corpuscular blood components in dependency from the pressures generated, and determines the biocompatibility of the procedure. A well-chosen set up respects the balance between invasiveness and need. According to the treatment goals, it might be appropriate to roughly categorize high-flow ECMO (full-blown) systems with blood flows of 4 L that offer more oxygenation and extensive CO_2 removal, mid-range flow systems with up to 2 L of blood flow (less oxygenation and good CO_2 removal), and low-flow systems up to 1 L of blood flow (no oxygenation benefit but significant CO_2 removal). Set-ups in these flow categories have been and are extensively used for numerous indications (**Tables 1** and **2**). In summary, for the classical rescue indication aimed primarily at assuring oxygenation, full-blown ECMO is indicated; for lung protection and reduced risk of mechanical ventilation, mid- and low blood flow devices are suitable.

In the following discussion, the authors describe the indications for which extracorporeal gas exchange is actually applied and critically reflect upon the current evidence justifying its use for each of these indications.

Table 1
Rationales for extracorporeal gas exchange use

	High Flow	Mid and Low Flow
Aim	Improving oxygenation and/or CO_2 elimination at critical thresholds	Reducing invasiveness of MV (TV, pressures, frequency, driving pressure, mechanical power)
Approach	Symptom oriented	Prevention oriented
Open questions	When and if needed how much supply is needed	Critical threshold where benefits outweigh risks
Control of success	Effect visible and in vivo measurable	Effect hypothetical and in vivo not verifiable

EVIDENCE AND INDICATIONS FOR MID- TO HIGH-FLOW EXTRACORPOREAL GAS EXCHANGE

Two randomized controlled trials in adult patients were performed some decades ago. The first multicenter study using ECMO for adult respiratory failure was published in 1979 and demonstrated no survival benefit.[5] ECMO as a treatment option for acute respiratory failure in the adult was carefully revised by Gattinoni and colleagues,[6] separating oxygenation and CO_2 removal with the conceptual innovation of preferentially using the ECMO unit for CO_2 removal. This approach set up the VV mode as standard of care for respiratory failure. Consequently, the second monocentric ECMO study (published in 1994) used the VV mode; however, this study also did not show outcome benefits for ECMO-treated patients.[7] Apart from many other aspects, such as approach- and device-related complications, one potential explanation for the lack of benefit is the lack of lung-protective ventilation.

In 2009, the CESAR trial was published.[8] In this randomized controlled trial, ARDS patients either continued to be treated conventionally in the hospital where they were randomized or transferred to 1 single ECMO center. There was a significant 6-month survival without disability benefit for patients predominantly treated with ECMO (37% vs 53%, $P = .03$) in the referral center. The study has been discussed. Although patients in the control group stayed in the participating hospitals without receiving a standardized protocol of lung-protective ventilation, the treatment group was transferred to an experienced ARDS and ECMO center. Twenty-two patients randomized to the ECMO-group did not receive ECMO but were treated conventionally or died during transport. In conclusion, for many (but mostly methodological) reasons, the

Table 2
Flow ranges and direction

Flow and Direction	Effect	Goal
Low flow systems <1000 mL VV	Limited CO_2 removal	Protective ventilation (VILI), reduction of delta pressure and/or mechanical power pH normalization
Midrange flow systems <2000 mL VV or AV	CO_2 elimination up to CO_2 minute Production limited oxygenation	Further reduction of ventilatory settings (VILI), marginal improvement of oxygenation
High-flow systems >4000 mL VV	Oxygenation and CO_2 removal	Assurance of oxygenation and CO_2 removal

2 negative trials did not kill the clinical use of ECMO, and the single positive trial did not further promote it. The ongoing successful use of ECMO in neonates and the acceptance of VV-ECMO as a rescue therapy in severe hypoxemic patients kept adult ECMO alive, with some centers remaining even highly active over the years.[9,10] In 2009, the worldwide influenza A H1N1 pandemic produced numerous patients with severe hypoxemic failure. The chest radiographs, computed tomography CT scans, and respiratory mechanics of many of these patients suggested a quasi cannot ventilate situation.[11] An observational study comparing severe ARDS cases caused by H1N1 influenza treated with VV-ECMO against a matched non-ECMO series of patients from a national registry showed a significantly reduced hospital mortality rate of 24% versus 47% (P>.001).[12,13] A systematic analysis of 4 studies found unclear benefit on hospital mortality, and a meta-analysis including the old ECMO study came more or less to the same conclusion.[14,15] However, although the overall evidence for the use of ECMO is limited and only supports its use as a rescue therapy, the H1N1 pandemic induced a revival of enthusiasm for ECMO that led worldwide to an explosion in the application of extracorporeal gas exchange techniques that still continues. The results of the multicenter EOLIA trial comparing ECMO with conventional treatment in adult patients with moderate ARDS according to the Berlin criteria plus at least 1 of 3 defined additional severity criteria will be available in 2018. However, this study was planned to seek an absolute mortality reduction of 20% between the study arms, a number that strongly reduces the likelihood of a positive result in the lung protection era.

Based on the current evidence, a German S3 guideline that was recently published recommended the use of (high-flow) ECMO only as a rescue therapy in patients with severe acute respiratory failure when all conservative strategies such as prone positioning have failed, and no sufficient oxygenation can be achieved. A weak recommendation (to be considered) is suggested for patients with acute respiratory insufficiency and refractory hypercapnia with profound acidosis.[16]

Interestingly, the authors of the guideline based the use of ECMO on structural requirements and strongly recommend a profound expertise in ARDS treatment, recommending that ECMO should only be provided in a center that regularly treats a minimum of 20 VV-ECMO cases per year.[16]

Structural requirements for the application of high-flow ECMO are based on expert opinion, because there is no clear evidence supporting this approach. However, the enthusiastic deployment of ECMO in Germany, where extracorporeal gas exchange is extensively used[17] (even in small hospitals that lack a sufficient number of ARDS patients per year) presents considerable risk for the patient. The structural requirements for centers recommended by the German guideline are in line with the position paper from the ECMOnet[18]:

- Extensive experience in the therapy of patients with severe ARDS
- Availability of a team (physicians and nurses) adequately trained and competent in the use of ECMO, 24 h/d
- A nurse-to-patient ratio that can be adapted to actual workload
- Sufficient support from blood bank, clinical laboratories, and radiology 24 h/d
- Vascular, abdominal and thoracic surgery directly available in case of an emergency
- Renal replacement therapy, bronchoscopy, echocardiography routinely available
- Structured educational program and training for the ECMO team
- An infrastructure that allows for the 24 h/d provision of care for patients with severe ARDS

- Safe and efficient transfer from referring hospitals
- Quality control and participation in national registries

EVIDENCE AND INDICATIONS FOR LOW FLOW EXTRACORPOREAL GAS EXCHANGE

As with high-flow VV-ECMO, low flow extracorporeal gas exchange is usually performed by pump-driven veno-venous access. Additionally, but less commonly used, there are also passive arteriovenous systems, driven by the natural arteriovenous pressure gradient. There are studies investigating CO_2 elimination using CO_2 dialysis by bicarbonate ultrafiltration and adjunctive techniques (like electro dialysis); however, their potential clinical relevance has to be further elucidated.[19–22]

A series of more recent prospective and retrospective studies showed that low-flow extracorporeal gas exchange ($ECCO_2R$) enables significant reduction of arterial CO_2 and leads to a marked pH increase. The amount of CO_2 eliminated by $ECCO_2R$ differs among the different systems and ranges usually between 20% and 50% of the patients' endogenous CO_2 production. The efficiency of extracorporeal CO_2 removal also depends on the CO_2 load. Knowledge of the capabilities of the system is important, because in hypercapnic respiratory failure with severe respiratory acidosis, the amount of CO_2 removal needed to enable lung protective ventilation or to support noninvasive ventilation-based avoidance of intubation might easily reach 50% to 60% of the total CO_2 production.

Most relevant clinical applications for low-flow extracorporeal gas exchange or better stated, extracorporeal CO_2 removal ($ECCO_2R$) are

- The avoidance of intubation in acute hypercapnic respiratory failure
- The reduction of the intensity of mechanical ventilation and prevention of ventilator-induced lung injury (VILI) in ARDS
- The shortening of invasive ventilation or facilitation of weaning in hypercapnic respiratory failure

A further indication might be use of these techniques as a bridge to lung transplantation.

LOW-FLOW EXTRACORPOREAL GAS EXCHANGE TO AVOID INTUBATION IN ACUTE RESPIRATORY FAILURE

In hypercapnic respiratory failure, the standard therapy for the failing respiratory muscles is the establishment of noninvasive, or, if unsuccessful, invasive ventilatory assistance. During recent years, $ECCO_2R$ evolved into a state where it is increasingly used as treatment option for patients with acute severe hypercapnic respiratory failure. The successful avoidance of intubation by $ECCO_2R$ in a patient with severe asthma was first described by Schneider.[23] Several recent case-control studies in severely exacerbated chronic obstructive pulmonary disease (COPD) patients demonstrated that intubation rates are reduced by the application of $ECCO_2R$. In 21 patients with COPD where NIV failed, the use of $ECCO_2R$ via pumpless AV extracorporeal gas exchange resulted in improved $PaCO_2$ and pH and the avoidance of intubation in 90% of the patients treated.[24] Retrospective comparison with a control group showed no significant difference in mortality at 28 days (19% vs 24%) or in the median lengths of stay in the intensive care unit (ICU) or hospital. Del Sorbo and colleagues[25] demonstrated a sufficient recompensation in 25 COPD patients when $ECCO_2R$ and NIV were combined and a reduced need for intubation when compared with a historical control group. Kluge and colleagues[26] were able to avoid invasive ventilation in 56% of cases treated with $ECCO_2R$, and Morelli and colleagues[27] prevented repeat intubation in 27 out of 30

COPD patients after failing NIV. However, it should also be noted that the recent study by Kluge and colleagues[26] reported a significant higher incidence of complications.

$ECCO_2R$ offers an attractive potential option, the avoidance of intubation in patients for whom intubation increases markedly their mortality risk. With the data currently available, it seems too early to recommend $ECCO_2R$ in combination with NIV as a technique to avoid intubation or as single therapeutic measure for patients with hypercapnic respiratory failure. There is a clear need for studies and trials that provide solid data on clinical relevance (ie, the risks and benefits of $ECCO_2R$ when the main objective is to avoid intubation).

LOW-FLOW EXTRACORPOREAL GAS EXCHANGE TO FACILITATE LUNG-PROTECTIVE VENTILATION

Avoidance or reduction of ventilator and ventilation-induced lung injury has become the holy grail during mechanical ventilation and weaning. Yet, it is not really known when and how much mechanical stressors generated either by externally applied forces or by breathing efforts of the patients lead to relevant pathologic changes of the lungs that exceed the innate repair mechanisms of the pulmonary matrix. However, as mechanical power applied during mechanical ventilation is spent to move and retain sufficient gas in the lungs that ensures adequate gas exchange, it is evident that adding the capabilities of an external gas exchanger will allow one to reduce the energy required in proportion to the oxygen and CO_2 transfer realized by the oxygenator. A series of prospective case-control studies have proven that $ECCO_2R$ can be used to reduce the invasiveness of mechanical ventilation by eliminating CO_2 and increasing pH.[28] In a recent meta-analysis, 14 studies with pumpless and pump-driven $ECCO_2R$ were included.[29] Although the capability of CO_2 removal could be confirmed, there was no effect on mortality or clinically relevant outcome measures. A further meta-analysis on COPD patients included 10 smaller case series[30] did not reveal positive effects on outcome (length of mechanical ventilation or survival) but demonstrated an increased rate of complications. The only multicenter randomized controlled trial by Bein[31] compared an ultraprotective ventilation strategy (3 mL/kg IBW) enabled by AV-$ECCO_2R$ with a conventional lung-protective approach. Results demonstrated significant effects on minute ventilation and delta pressure in the intervention group, and patients could be switched earlier to spontaneous breathing. Overall there was no difference with regard to mortality or ventilator-free days, but a post hoc subgroup analysis revealed a benefit for the more severe cases ($Pa_{O_2}/Fi_{O_2} < 150$ mm Hg) included in the study.

LOW-FLOW EXTRACORPOREAL GAS EXCHANGE TO FACILITATE WEANING

For patients during difficult or prolonged weaning it seems feasible that the use of $ECCO_2R$ might facilitate weaning from mechanical ventilation or replace ventilation completely. The potential advantages, if compared with a prolonged process of invasive ventilation, are the avoidance of ventilator-associated complications and improved patient comfort. However, the potential advantages of replacing mechanical ventilation need to be weighed against the complications of the procedure. Although low-flow $ECCO_2R$ requires vascular access with smaller venous cannulas when compared with high-flow ECMO, vascular injury, the need for therapeutic anticoagulation, and the risk of bleedings and thromboembolic complications cannot be ignored. In 2007, Elliot[32] reported 2 patients suffering from life-threatening asthma in whom pumpless $ECCO_2R$ added to invasive mechanical ventilation with IMV ensured adequate gas exchange by correction of hypercapnia and acidosis, and then facilitated weaning from mechanical ventilation. Burki and colleagues[33] used

$ECCO_2R$ in a low-flow range for 11 patients being ventilated invasively and were able to successfully support weaning in three 3 patients and to reduce ventilatory support in another 3 patients. Successful facilitation of weaning was also reported in 5 patients with COPD and acute respiratory acidosis by Abrams, who used a midflow device for $ECCO_2R$.[34] All patients survived to hospital discharge.

Before broadly introducing $ECCO_2R$ to support weaning into the clinical routine, there is a serious need for studies with regards to short- and long-term outcome measures. Currently, there is an ongoing pilot study on the use of extracorporeal CO_2 removal during the weaning process from mechanical ventilation (ClinicalTrials.gov; NCT02259335, WeanPRO) that will add further knowledge, but more trials are needed.

ACTUAL STATUS AND OUTLOOK

Having described the indications for which extracorporeal gas exchange is actually applied alongside the low-to-nonexistent evidence for its benefits in each of these indications, the worldwide enthusiastic deployment raises serious questions. The beneficial effects of prone positioning have been clearly demonstrated; however, not more than 31% of patients going on extracorporeal support have been placed prone beforehand.[35] The use of prone position in ARDS patients in general is alarmingly low.[36] Instead, an expensive, resource-consuming technique for which–at least so far–serious evidence is lacking is increasingly being used. There is certainly no single or simple explanation for this striking fact; however, for obvious reasons, improved quality of care seems not to be the key driver. Most of the indications for which extracorporeal gas exchange techniques are now used still represent experimental medicine. There are good reasons to assume that financial interests, and reimbursement, fascination to deal with new gadgets, and personal ambition play a much greater role than physicians might believe or wish to acknowledge.[37] It seems reasonable to use a technique that theoretically allows us to reduce the occurrence of VILI; however, first it is not really known at which threshold mechanical forces applied to the lungs become clinically relevant and, second ECMO is by far not without own risks. Most relevant adverse effects are bleeding (with intracranial bleeding being the most fatal one), thrombosis, limb ischemia, and vascular injuries.[38,39] So balancing risks and benefits of MV and extracorporeal gas exchange while describing thresholds where the potential benefits of one procedure are outweighed by its adverse effects will be crucial to define the role of extracorporeal support in the future when prevention and/or a further promotion of lung injury is the aim. The rationale for the classic rescue indication is obvious. Avoiding severe, life-threatening hypoxemia needs no further reasoning. Yet, it is not really known the individual critical hypoxemia thresholds, and the evident risks of applied treatments to prevent it create other considerations compared with the prevention of VILI.[40]

Also, ECMO is worldwide very likely used with the intention to replace at least in part the gas exchange via the native lungs. However, with the currently applied technologies physicians have little idea regarding how much of this gas exchange is realized via the native lungs and which amount of gas exchange is provided by the membrane lung. It is not even known how much CO_2 is removed in total per unit time interval or what is going to happen physiologically if one shifts, by changing settings, the partitioning of gas exchange between native lung and oxygenator. For example, increasing the oxygen transfer via the membrane lung might reduce hypoxemic pulmonary vasoconstriction and consecutively lead to a lower arterial oxygen partial pressure. Currently physicians simply turn 2 knobs; they largely miss the complex consequences and interactions and follow surrogates who do not allow them to carefully assess if they are doing the right things. To technically implement extracorporeal gas exchange is relatively simple; however, because it deeply influences physiology and pathophysiology, prudent use of this technology requires understanding and better monitoring that allows observing and following the interaction between extracorporeal support and native lungs.

Extracorporeal gas exchange as currently implemented unquestionably is a powerful tool. Technical developments will certainly further improve the gas exchange capabilities and reduce risks and adverse effects. It opens a wide spectrum of potentially beneficial indications that might lead to better care for patients in need. However, to give extracorporeal gas exchange a fair chance for a bright future one needs understanding, careful monitoring with better technologies, physiologic and observational studies, and patience to avoid a fallback to the times before the H1N1 stimulus by multicenter studies that fail to show benefits, as has happened in many other studies in intensive care medicine.

REFERENCES

1. Gattinoni L, Tonetti T, Cressoni M, et al. Ventilator-related causes of lung injury: the mechanical power. Intensive Care Med 2016;42:1567–75.
2. Clowes GH Jr, Hopkins AL, Neville WE. An artificial lung dependent upon diffusion of oxygen and carbon dioxide through plastic membranes. J Thorac Surg 1956;32:630–7.
3. Hill JD, De Leval MR, Fallat RJ, et al. Acute respiratory insufficiency: treatment with prolonged extracorporeal oxygenation. J Thorac Cardiovasc Surg 1972;64: 551–62.
4. Bartlett RH. Esperanza: presidential address. Trans Am Soc Artif Intern Organs 1985;31:723–6.
5. Zapol WM, Snider MT, Hill JD, et al. Extracorporeal membrane oxygenation in severe acute respiratory failure: a randomized prospective study. JAMA 1979;242: 2193–6.
6. Gattinoni L, Kolobow T, Damia G, et al. Extracorporeal carbon dioxide removal (ECCO2R): a new form of respiratory assistance. Int J Artif Organs 1979;2:183–5.
7. Morris AH, Wallace CJ, Menlove RL, et al. Randomized clinical trial of pressure-controlled inverse ratio ventilation and extracorporeal CO2 removal for adult respiratory distress syndrome. Am J Respir Crit Care Med 1994;149:295–305.
8. Peek GJ, Mugford M, Tiruvoipati R, et al, CESAR trial collaboration. Efficacy and economic assessment of conventional ventilatory support versus extracorporeal membrane oxygenation for severe adult respiratory failure (CESAR): a multicentre randomised controlled trial. Lancet 2009;374:1351–63.
9. UK Collaborative ECMO Trail Group: UK collaborative randomised trial of neonatal extracorporeal membrane oxygenation. Lancet 1996;348:75–82.
10. Bartlett RH, Roloff DW, Custer JR, et al. Extracorporeal life support: the University of Michigan experience. JAMA 2000;283:904–8.
11. Australia and New Zealand Extracorporeal Membrane Oxygenation (ANZ ECMO) Influenza Investigators, Davies A, Jones D, Bailey M, et al. Extracorporeal membrane oxygenation for 2009 influenza A(H1N1) acute respiratory distress syndrome. JAMA 2009;302:1888–95.
12. Noah MA, Peek GJ, Finney SJ, et al. Referral to an extracorporeal membrane oxygenation center and mortality among patients with severe 2009 influenza A(H1N1). JAMA 2011;306:1659–68.
13. Pham T, Combes A, Rozé H, et al, REVA Research Network. Extracorporeal membrane oxygenation for pandemic influenza a(h1n1)-induced acute respiratory

distress syndrome a cohort study and propensity-matched analysis. Am J Respir Crit Care Med 2013;187(3):276–85.

14. Tramm R, Ilic D, Davies AR, et al. Extracorporeal membrane oxygenation for critically ill adults. Cochrane Database Syst Rev 2015;(1):CD010381.

15. Zampieri FG, Mendes PV, Ranzani OT, et al. Extracorporeal membrane oxygenation for severe respiratory failure in adult patients: a systematic review and meta-analysis of current evidence. A systematic review and meta-analysis of current evidence. J Crit Care 2013;28:998–1005.

16. S3-Leitlinie"Invasive Beatmung und Einsatz extrakorporaler Verfahren bei akuter respiratorischer Insuffizienz." Available at: http://www.awmf.org/leitlinien/detail/ll/001-021.html.

17. Karagiannidis C, Brodie D, Strassmann S, et al. Extracorporeal membrane oxygenation: evolving epidemiology and mortality. Intensive Care Med 2016;42:889–96.

18. Combes A, Brodie D, Bartlett R, et al, International ECMO Network (ECMONet). Position paper for the organization of extracorporeal membrane oxygenation programs for acute respiratory failure in adult patients. Am J Respir Crit Care Med 2014;190:488–96.

19. Moerer O, Quintel M. Protective and ultra-protective ventilation: using pumpless interventional lung assist (iLA). Minerva Anestesiol 2011;77:537–44.

20. Allardet-Servent J, Castanier M, Signouret T, et al. Safety and efficacy of combined extracorporeal CO2 removal and renal replacement therapy in patients with acute respiratory distress syndrome and acute kidney injury: the pulmonary and renal support in acute respiratory distress syndrome study. Crit Care Med 2015;43:2570–81.

21. Cressoni M, Zanella A, Epp M, et al. Decreasing pulmonary ventilation through bicarbonate ultrafiltration: an experimental study. Crit Care Med 2009;37:2612–8.

22. Zanella A, Castagna L, Salerno D, et al. Respiratory electrodialysis. A novel, highly efficient extracorporeal CO2 removal technique. Am J Respir Crit Care Med 2015;192:719–26.

23. Schneider TM, Bence T, Brettner F. "Awake" ECCO2R superseded intubation in a near-fatal asthma attack. J Intensive Care 2017;5:53.

24. Braune S, Sieweke A, Brettner F, et al. The feasibility and safety of extracorporeal carbon dioxide removal to avoid intubation in patients with COPD unresponsive to noninvasive ventilation for acute hypercapnic respiratory failure (ECLAIR study): multicentre case-control study. Intensive Care Med 2016;42:1437–44.

25. Del Sorbo L, Pisani L, Filippini C, et al. Extracorporeal CO2 removal in hypercapnic patients at risk of noninvasive ventilation failure: a matched cohort study with historical control. Crit Care Med 2015;43:120–7.

26. Kluge S, Braune SA, Engel M, et al. Avoiding invasive mechanical ventilation by extracorporeal carbon dioxide removal in patients failing noninvasive ventilation. Intensive Care Med 2012;38:1632–9.

27. Morelli A, Del Sorbo L, Pesenti A, et al. Extracorporeal carbon dioxide removal (ECCO2R) in patients with acute respiratory failure. Intensive Care Med 2017;43:519–30.

28. Fanelli V, Ranieri MV, Mancebo J, et al. Feasibility and safety of low-flow extracorporeal carbon dioxide removal to facilitate ultra-protective ventilation in patients with moderate acute respiratory distress syndrome. Crit Care 2016;20:36.

29. Fitzgerald M, Millar J, Blackwood B, et al. Extracorporeal carbon dioxide removal for patients with acute respiratory failure secondary to the acute respiratory distress syndrome: a systematic review. Crit Care 2014;18(3):222.

30. Sklar MC, Beloncle F, Katsios CM, et al. Extracorporeal carbon dioxide removal in patients with chronic obstructive pulmonary disease: a systematic review. Intensive Care Med 2015;41:1752–62.

31. Bein T, Weber-Carstens S, Goldmann A, et al. Lower tidal volume strategy ($\approx$ 3 ml/kg) combined with extracorporeal CO_2 removal versus 'conventional' protective ventilation (6 ml/kg) in severe ARDS: the prospective randomized Xtravent-study. Intensive Care Med 2013;39:847–56.

32. Elliot SC, Paramasivam K, Oram J, et al. Pumpless extracorporeal carbon dioxide removal for life-threatening asthma. Crit Care Med 2007;35:945–8.

33. Burki NK, Mani RK, Herth FJF, et al. A novel extracorporeal CO_2 removal system: results of a pilot study of hypercapnic respiratory failure in patients with COPD. Chest 2013;143:678–86.

34. Abrams DC, Brenner K, Burkart KM, et al. Pilot study of extracorporeal carbon dioxide removal to facilitate extubation and ambulation in exacerbations of chronic obstructive pulmonary disease. Ann Am Thorac Soc 2013;10:307–14.

35. Li X, Scales DC, Kavanagh BP. Unproven and expensive before proven and cheap: extracorporeal membrane oxygenation versus prone position in acute respiratory distress syndrome. Am J Respir Crit Care Med 2018;197(8):991–3.

36. Guérin C, Beuret P, Constantin JM, et al, investigators of the APRONET Study Group, the REVA Network, the Réseau recherche de la Société Française d'Anesthésie-Réanimation (SFAR-recherche) and the ESICM Trials Group. A prospective international observational prevalence study on prone positioning of ARDS patients: the APRONET (ARDS Prone Position Network) study. Intensive Care Med 2018;44:22–37.

37. Quintel M, Gattinoni L, Weber-Carstens S. The German ECMO inflation: when things other than health and care begin to rule medicine. Intensive Care Med 2016;42:1264–6.

38. Menaker J, Tabatabai A, Rector R, et al. Incidence of cannula-associated deep vein thrombosis after veno-venous extracorporeal membrane oxygenation. ASAIO J 2017;63:588–91.

39. Klinzing S, Wenger U, Stretti F, et al. Neurologic injury with severe adult respiratory distress syndrome in patients undergoing extracorporeal membrane oxygenation: a single-center retrospective analysis. Anesth Analg 2017;125:1544–8.

40. Gattinoni L, Marini JJ, Quintel M. Time to rethink the approach to treating acute respiratory distress syndrome. JAMA 2018;319:664–6.

Section II: Ventricular Assist Devices

Preface

Ventricular Assist Devices for Cardiogenic Shock and Advanced Chronic Heart Failure

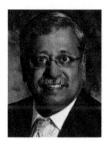

Srinivas Murali, MD
Editor

Over 6 million Americans suffer from heart failure (HF), and 900,000 new patients are diagnosed each year. Despite advances in medical therapy, 50% of HF patients die within 5 years of diagnosis. It is also the leading cause of hospitalization in the Medicare population; up to 20% of patients are rehospitalized within 30 days, and up to 30% are rehospitalized within 90 days of discharge from the hospital. The total cost of HF care exceeds 30 billion dollars annually, and this accounts for expenses related to all health care services, prescriptions, and missed days of work. About half of all HF patients have the phenotype of reduced left ventricular ejection fraction, while the remainder have preserved left ventricular ejection fraction.

Over 1 million HF patients have advanced chronic disease with disabling symptoms that are progressive despite optimal medical therapy. Many of these patients are critically ill and require careful hemodynamic monitoring in the intensive care unit during hospitalizations. Cardiac transplantation is an effective treatment for some of these patients who were suitable candidates. Unfortunately, this option is available to only 2500 patients annually because of a lack of availability of donor hearts. For the remaining patients, durable mechanical circulatory support with ventricular assist devices (VAD) is a viable option. Though the market for VAD therapy in advanced chronic HF has been estimated at 250,000 patients annually, presently only 3000 patients receive VAD implantation each year. As clinical outcomes on VAD therapy continue to improve and approach that seen with cardiac transplantation, it is anticipated that many more patients will receive this therapy in the future. Sound knowledge base in VAD is therefore very important for all health professionals who will be called upon to deliver care to this group of patients. This issue of *Critical Care Clinics* discusses in detail the use of VADs both in cardiogenic shock and in advanced chronic HF.

Crit Care Clin 34 (2018) xv–xvii
https://doi.org/10.1016/j.ccc.2018.04.002
0749-0704/18/© 2018 Published by Elsevier Inc.

criticalcare.theclinics.com

Cardiogenic shock is a form of acute advanced HF commonly caused by myocardial dysfunction from acute coronary syndrome. It is often associated with multiorgan system failure and carries an in-hospital mortality of 50% to 60%. Acute coronary revascularization, hemodynamic-guided tailored therapy, and timely use of percutaneous mechanical circulatory support devices are the mainstays of therapy today. More importantly, the complexity of care in these patients demands the deployment of multidisciplinary teams delivering care collaboratively in a coordinated manner within a tertiary care or quaternary care hospital environment to achieve the best clinical outcomes. A contemporary approach to targeted management of cardiogenic shock is described by Mithun Chakravarthy and coauthors in their article.

Contemporary chronic mechanical circulatory support mostly comprises durable left ventricular assist devices (LVADs). These devices unload the left ventricle and increase preload to the right ventricle, putting patients at risk for acute and/or chronic right ventricular failure, which can markedly diminish the short- and long-term benefit of device therapy. Chronic right ventricular failure in LVAD-supported patients not only decreases quality of life but also puts these patients at risk for frequent hospitalizations. Preventing right ventricular failure, recognizing it early should it develop, and treating it aggressively are therefore mandatory. This is described by Amresh Raina and his coauthor in their article.

The evolution in technology has increased expectations from LVAD therapy for both physicians and patients. It is simply not enough to maintain normal cardiac output and end-organ function at rest, but it is expected that these devices allow for appropriate augmentation of flow with activity to facilitate a good functional capacity and quality of life. Therefore, understanding the complex physiologic interaction between the LVAD and the native heart and vascular system is needed so that the device can be optimally programmed to deliver flow in each patient. Interrogation of device parameters, using them in the diagnosis of specific complications, and tailoring them as necessary are important in the management of patients on LVAD support. This is discussed in the article by Inna Tchoukina and her coauthors.

LVAD therapy is associated with significant risk to the patient. Early complications can include bleeding and right ventricular failure, while long-term complications are neurologic dysfunction related to ischemic or hemorrhagic stroke and device dysfunction or failure from thrombosis. Driveline and pocket infections can occur both early and late after device implantation. Flow characteristics within the device can result in hemocompatibility issues leading to gastrointestinal bleeding. Mitigating the risk of these complications by improved technologic design and novel surgical techniques; preventing right ventricular failure, better anticoagulation protocols, and optimal blood pressure control; and tailoring device parameters are required to achieve optimal long-term outcomes. The complications on durable LVAD support are described by the article by Sitaramesh Emani.

Despite the progress made over the past two decades, there still remain several challenges with left LVAD for advanced HF. The therapy is expensive; patients on device support utilize significant resources, and many remain a burden to their families and society. As the demand for this therapy grows by its adoption to chronic HF patients with less advanced disease, the health economic impact has to be addressed. Cost-effectiveness must be demonstrated by developing reliable risk prediction tools for selection of "ideal" patients, engaging in shared decision making, deploying multidisciplinary team-based care using pathways that minimize the threat of complications, and using aggressive cardiovascular rehabilitation. It is hoped that, in the future, patients on LVAD therapy will return to their communities as independent citizens ready for societal contributions. The challenges and future directions in LVAD therapy are discussed by Manreet Kanwar and coauthors in their article.

The comprehensive content in this issue is targeted toward cardiologists, cardiac surgeons, intensivists, and other critical care health professionals, who are either involved or likely to be involved in the care of advanced HF patients on VAD support. The articles are easy to read and full of practical information that is very relevant to patient care. I want to extend my very sincere and grateful appreciation to all the authors and coauthors for their outstanding work. All of them are experts in this field, and I had much pleasure working with them on this project. I would like to thank my parents, who are my role models and whose love and guidance are always with me in whatever I pursue. Most importantly, I wish to thank my loving and supportive wife, Marie, my three wonderful children, Vijay, Sara, and Rani, and my daughter-in-law, Margaux, who provide unending inspiration.

Srinivas Murali, MD
Division of Cardiovascular Medicine
Cardiovascular Institute
Drexel University College of Medicine
Allegheny Health Network
16th Floor, South Tower
320 East North Avenue
Pittsburgh, PA 15212, USA

E-mail address:
srinivas.murali@ahn.org

A Targeted Management Approach to Cardiogenic Shock

Mithun Chakravarthy, MD, Masaki Tsukashita, MD,
Srinivas Murali, MD*

KEYWORDS

- Cardiogenic shock • Hemodynamics • Temporary mechanical support
- Intraaortic balloon pump • Coronary revascularization

KEY POINTS

- Acute coronary syndrome remains the leading cause of cardiogenic shock. In-hospital mortality in cardiogenic shock ranges from 40% to 50%.
- Timely transfer to a tertiary or quaternary medical center with critical care management, mechanical circulatory support, and multidisciplinary team-based care is necessary to achieve good clinical outcomes.
- Coronary revascularization is the mainstay of treatment for cardiogenic shock. Aggressive, hemodynamically guided medical management with continuous assessment of hemodynamic goals and end-organ function is recommended.
- Mechanical circulatory support is often necessary. Multidisciplinary team-based decision making should drive the choice of mechanical support device and monitoring for need for escalation of therapy.
- Durable mechanical circulatory support may be necessary in suitable candidates once hemodynamic stabilization is achieved.

INTRODUCTION

Cardiogenic shock is a primary cardiac syndrome, characterized by a low cardiac output state that deranges cardiac homeostasis resulting in sustained tissue hypoperfusion (>30 minutes), a very high morbidity and in hospital mortality of more than 60%.[1] Clinical criteria include hypotension with a systolic blood pressure of less than 90 mm Hg or pharmacologic intervention or mechanical support to maintain systolic blood pressure of 90 mm Hg or greater, and cool extremities or multiorgan failure

Disclosures: None.
Cardiovascular Institute, Allegheny General Hospital, 320 East North Avenue, Pittsburgh, PA 15212, USA
* Corresponding author.
E-mail address: Srinivas.Murali@ahn.org

Crit Care Clin 34 (2018) 423–437
https://doi.org/10.1016/j.ccc.2018.03.009
0749-0704/18/© 2018 Elsevier Inc. All rights reserved.

characterized by urine output of 30 mL/h or less, mental status changes, and lactic acidosis. Although not required, hemodynamic measurements can help to diagnose cardiogenic shock. Hemodynamic criteria include a depressed cardiac index (≤ 2.2 L/min/m^2) and an elevated pulmonary capillary wedge pressure (PCWP) (≥ 15 mm Hg). Rapid diagnosis, timely referral to a tertiary or quaternary medical facility, and shared decision making among a multidisciplinary team of specialists including interventional cardiologists, advanced heart failure specialists, cardiac surgeons, and cardiac intensivists is needed to achieve the best clinical outcomes for every patient.[1] Despite advances in critical care management, reperfusion therapy, and mechanical circulatory support, mortality in cardiogenic shock remains frustratingly high.

ETIOLOGY

The etiologies of cardiogenic shock are listed in **Box 1**. The most common cause of cardiogenic shock, affecting more than 80% of the patients is myocardial dysfunction from acute myocardial infarction with loss of at least 40% of left ventricular (LV) mass or loss of less than 40% LV mass with recurrent, sustained, and refractory ventricular arrhythmias. The prevalence of cardiogenic shock from acute myocardial infarction has continued to increase over the past decade with no change in clinical outcomes. Coexistent or isolated right ventricular (RV) infarction or development of mechanical complications such as papillary muscle rupture with acute mitral regurgitation, LV free wall rupture, or acute ventricular septal defect frequently results in cardiogenic shock. It remains the leading cause of in-hospital mortality after an acute myocardial infarction. Other disorders leading to severe impairment of myocardial function such as acute decompensation of chronic heart failure, acute myocarditis, peripartum cardiomyopathy, or stress-induced Takotsubo cardiomyopathy can result in cardiogenic

---

Box 1
Etiology of cardiogenic shock

A. Myocardial disease
- Acute myocardial infarction
  ○ Greater than 40% loss of LV mass
  ○ Less than 40% loss of LV mass with recurrent, refractory arrhythmia
  ○ RV infarction
  ○ Mechanical complication (papillary muscle or free wall rupture, VSD)
- Acute decompensated heart failure
  ○ Chronic heart failure with acute decompensation
  ○ Initial presentation of acute heart failure (myocarditis, peripartum CM, Takotsubo CM)
- Postcardiotomy shock
- Miscellaneous (dynamic LVOT obstruction, myocardial depression in sepsis, myocardial contusion)

B. Valve disease
- Stenosis, regurgitation, or prosthetic valve failure

C. Electrical disease
- Bradyarrhythmia or atrial/ventricular tachyarrhythmia

D. Extracardiac disease
- Constrictive pericarditis, cardiac tamponade, pulmonary embolism

Abbreviations: CM, cardiomyopathy; LV, left ventricular; LVOT, left ventricular outflow tract; RV, right ventricular; VSD, ventral septal defect.

Table 1
Severity of cardiogenic shock

Parameter	Pre/Early Shock	Shock	Severe Shock
Systolic BP (mm Hg)	<100	<90	<90
Heart rate (bpm)	70–100	>100	>120
Extremities	Cool	Cool	Cool
Mental status	Normal	Altered	Obtunded
Blood lactate level (mmol/L)	Normal (<1.0)	>2.0	>4.0
Cardiac index (L/min/m^2)	>2.0	1.5–2.0	<1.5
PCWP (mm Hg)	<20	>20	>30
CPO (watts)	>1.0	<1.0	<0.6
VIS	<20	20–30	>30

Abbreviations: BP, blood pressure; CPO, cardiac power output (mean arterial pressure × cardiac output/451; mean arterial pressure is systolic BP - diastolic BP/3 + diastolic BP); VIS, vasoactive inotropic score (dopamine dose [μg/kg/min] + dobutamine dose [μg/kg/min] + 10 × milrinone dose [μg/kg/min] + 100 × epinephrine dose [μg/kg/min] + 10 × phenylephrine dose [μg/kg/min] + 100 × norepinephrine dose [μg/kg/min] + 10,000 × vasopressin dose [U/kg/min]).

shock. Valve disease, bradyarrhythmias and tachyarrhythmias, and extracardiac causes such as pericardial disease and pulmonary embolism can also cause cardiogenic shock.[1]

PATHOPHYSIOLOGY

The pathophysiology of cardiogenic shock involves a cascade of biologic events that begin with acute cardiac injury and spiral toward death (**Fig. 1**).[1] The decrease in cardiac output and stroke volume results in hypotension, decreased peripheral perfusion, and coronary ischemia. The resulting compensatory peripheral vasoconstriction increases afterload to the LV and further exacerbates myocardial dysfunction. Alternatively, a systemic inflammatory response triggered by the acute cardiac injury causes vasodilation by increasing circulating levels of nitric oxide, peroxy nitrite, and proinflammatory cytokines such as tumor necrosis factor-α and interleukins. These mediators further decrease cardiac output and stroke volume by impairing contractility. Myocardial dysfunction also increases LV end-diastolic pressure causing pulmonary edema and hypoxia, which can further exacerbate myocardial ischemia.

All hemodynamic phenotypes of cardiogenic shock are characterized by a low cardiac index. However, based on which pathobiologic phenomenon is dominant, the PCWP is either increased or normal, and the systemic vascular resistance is either high or low. The classic cardiogenic shock phenotype, which is seen in more than two-thirds of patients, is characterized by a low cardiac index, high PCWP, and a high systemic vascular resistance. The euvolemic cardiogenic shock phenotype, which is typically seen with RV infarction, has a low cardiac index, high systemic vascular resistance, and a normal PCWP. Finally, the vasodilatory cardiogenic shock phenotype has a low cardiac index, low systemic vascular resistance, and a high PCWP. Bedside hemodynamic monitoring can help to precisely identify the hemodynamic phenotype of the patient.[1]

EVALUATION OF A PATIENT IN CARDIOGENIC SHOCK

More than 80% of patients with cardiogenic shock have acute coronary syndrome, which should be promptly diagnosed with an electrocardiogram and measurement

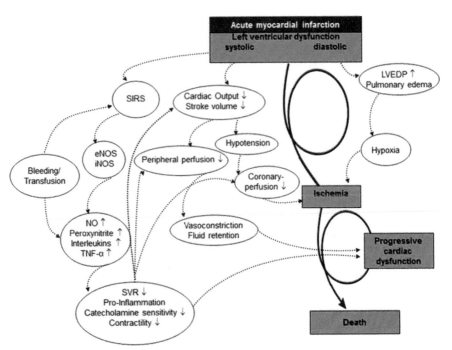

Fig. 1. Pathophysiology of cardiogenic shock. The myocardial dysfunction starts a cascade of biologic events that result in progressive cardiac dysfunction and death. eNOS, endothelial nitric oxide synthase; iNOS, inducible nitric oxide synthase; LVEDP, left ventricular end-diastolic pressure; NO, nitric oxide; SIRS, systemic inflammatory response syndrome; SVR, systemic vascular resistance; TNF-α, tumor necrosis factor alpha.

of cardiac troponins. Bedside echocardiography can help to define the extent of myocardial damage, evaluate for valve disease, and diagnose complications such as papillary muscle rupture, free wall rupture, or ventricular septal defect. Continuous bedside hemodynamic monitoring is often necessary to define the hemodynamic phenotype and track response to medical management.[1] Serial measurements of blood lactate level and arterial blood gas measurement are particularly helpful to diagnose metabolic and respiratory acid–base alterations and monitor progress and response to therapeutic interventions. Routine laboratory evaluation to assess renal and hepatic function will help with the recognition of dysfunction in these target organs. Acute kidney injury, which occurs from renal hypoperfusion, is associated with an increase in serum creatinine and decrease in urine output, and often results in worse outcomes. Acute ischemic or congestive liver injury can occur in cardiogenic shock and is associated with elevated liver enzymes, serum bilirubin, and prothrombin time.

RISK STRATIFICATION AND CLINICAL OUTCOMES

A composite of clinical findings, hemodynamic parameters, and level of pharmacologic support is often used to categorize the severity of cardiogenic shock (**Table 1**).[2,3] In-hospital mortality rates in cardiogenic shock have not changed in the past decade and remain between 50% and 60%. Risk factors for mortality include older age, female gender, prior history of hypertension, diabetes mellitus, ST segment elevation myocardial infarction, and heart failure. Multivessel coronary artery disease and anterior wall ST segment elevation myocardial infarction, particularly those associated with new left bundle branch block, are also risk factors for poor outcomes.[4]

A number of risk stratification tools have been proposed in cardiogenic shock. Some of the tools were derived from critically ill patients in a general intensive care unit. The APACHE II (Acute Physiology and Chronic Health Evaluation) score is derived from 13 variables obtained in the first 24 hours of admission to an intensive care unit.[5] The recently described APACHE III score adds additional variables including gender, race, etiology of shock, and comorbidities.[6] The SAPS II (Simplified Acute Physiology Score) score includes 12 physiologic variables.[7] These scores can predict in hospital mortality with reasonable discrimination. The CardShock score was derived by European investigators from 219 patients with cardiogenic shock and uses 7 variables, each of which individually predicts in-hospital mortality (**Table 2**). The score ranges from 0 to 9, and is highly sensitive with an area under the curve of 0.83. The in-hospital mortality risk increases with the score, and patients with a score of 9 have 100% mortality. This score requires further external validation in greater number of patients.[8]

According to the American Heart Association consensus statement on cardiogenic shock, clinical outcomes can be improved with management of these patients in a cardiac intensive care unit located within a tertiary or quaternary medical center with on-site monitoring, medical services, and therapeutic technologies that allow for coordination and delivery of multidisciplinary team based care.[1] A proposed model is one where a cardiogenic shock team that includes specialists in interventional cardiology, advanced heart failure and cardiac surgery is activated upon diagnosis (**Fig. 2**). The team follows a clinical pathway for risk stratification and management while carefully monitoring progress and working collaboratively to ensure timely decision making pertaining to revascularization and the use of interventions for circulatory support. Although such a team-based approach can improve the likelihood of survival

Table 2
CardioShock risk score

Variable	Points
Age >75 y	1
Confusion at presentation	1
Prior MI or CABG	1
Acute coronary syndrome	1
LVEF <40%	1
Blood lactate level (mmol/L)	
<2	0
2–4	1
>4	2
Glomerular filtration rate (mL/min)	
>60	0
30–60	1
>60	2
Maximum points	9

Abbreviations: CABG, coronary artery bypass grafting; LVEF, left ventricular ejection fraction; MI, myocardial infarction.

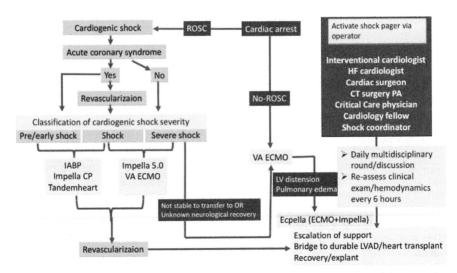

Fig. 2. Proposed model for a cardiogenic shock program. This proposed model summarizes the role of a multidisciplinary shock team in the diagnosis and classification of the severity of cardiogenic shock and timely decision making regarding medical management as well as temporary percutaneous and surgical mechanical circulatory support. IABP, intraaortic balloon pump; LVAD, left ventricular assist device; ROSC, return of spontaneous circulation; VA-ECMO, venoarterial extracorporeal membrane oxygenation.

to discharge from the hospital, the implementation of such systems of care can be challenging. Standardizing requirements for tertiary and quaternary treatment centers that not only include capabilities for temporary and durable mechanical circulatory support, but also triage decisions, care coordination, resource allocation for transport teams, and team-based care are necessary to manage costs and achieve best clinical outcomes.

TREATMENT
Coronary Revascularization

Coronary revascularization remains the mainstay of treatment for patients with acute coronary syndrome and cardiogenic shock. Guidelines recommend early invasive strategy with percutaneous coronary intervention or coronary artery bypass grafting for all patients with acute coronary syndrome and cardiogenic shock, regardless of the time from the onset of myocardial damage and even in the presence of uncertain neurologic status or prior administration of fibrinolytic therapy. Revascularization of both the culprit vessel as well any other nonculprit, hemodynamically significant stenosis is recommended. However, a recent large multicenter trial that enrolled patients who had multi-vessel coronary artery disease and acute myocardial infarction with cardiogenic shock, the 30-day risk of a composite of death or severe renal failure leading to renal-replacement therapy was lower among those who initially underwent PCI of the culprit lesion only than among those who underwent immediate multi-vessel PCI.[9] After percutaneous coronary intervention dual antiplatelet therapy should be administered as long as there are no bleeding complications. If oral agents cannot be administered, intravenous glycoprotein IIb/IIIa inhibitors should be considered.[10,11]

Pharmacologic Therapy for Hemodynamic Support

Hemodynamic monitoring is recommended in all patients and once baseline data are available, hemodynamic goals must be established. Inotropic agents like dopamine, dobutamine, milrinone or epinephrine should be used alone or in combination to normalize the cardiac index. Hypotension, if present despite inotropic therapy, should be treated with vasoactive agents such as vasopressin, phenylephrine, or norepinephrine used alone or in combination. Blood pressure, heart rate, oxygenation, and end-organ function including urine output, and mental status must be monitored closely. In addition to the cardiac index, central venous pressures, pulmonary artery pressures, PCWP, and systemic vascular resistance should be monitored hourly, and blood lactate level, glomerular filtration rate, and cardiac power output (CPO) every 6 hours. Ancillary measures such as stress ulcer prophylaxis and deep vein thrombosis prophylaxis should be prescribed. If the patient is mechanically ventilated, appropriate evidence-based management of ventilation and oxygenation is required. Renal replacement therapy should be considered in those with severe acute kidney injury and poor urine output. The hemodynamic goals should be revisited every 6 hours and medical management should be titrated as necessary. Patients who are not responding to medical management and fail to achieve hemodynamic goals should be considered for mechanical circulatory support. Appropriate timing of mechanical circulatory support is crucial to achieving good clinical outcomes and the choice of support is based on the severity of shock.[1]

Temporary Percutaneous Left Ventricular Mechanical Support Devices

Temporary mechanical support devices include pulsatile pumps (intraaortic balloon pump [IABP]), the left ventricle to aorta axial pumps (transvalvular device; Impella 2.5 and CP; Abiomed Inc, Danvers, MA), left atrium to femoral artery pump (TandemHeart; CardiacAssist Inc, Pittsburgh, PA), and the right atrium or central vein to a systemic artery pump with oxygenation (venoarterial extracorporeal membrane oxygenation).[12] An ideal temporary mechanical support device should improve the mean arterial pressure and cardiac output, and thus the CPO. CPO has shown to be an independent predictor of mortality in the setting of cardiogenic shock. In addition, the device should be easily available, easy to deploy, and should have minimal complications.[13]

The identification of cardiogenic shock and defining the level of shock can guide one to select the device needed to provide adequate hemodynamic support. Selection of the device primarily depends on the level of support needed (presumed hemodynamic support it provides), and on the patient's clinical characteristics like presence of peripheral vascular disease. Operator expertise, product availability, and other technical challenges also play a role in device selection. The devices available are compared in **Table 3**.

Intraaortic balloon pump

The IABP has been in use for almost 5 decades, and is the most commonly used device for temporary mechanical circulatory support. It unloads the left ventricle and decreases the afterload by creating a suction-like phenomenon, thereby decreasing myocardial oxygen demand. Most important, it also increases coronary perfusion during diastole by displacement of blood. However, its effect on cardiac output and CPO is minimal and it is not an ideal device for patients in severe or profound cardiogenic shock.[14]

The IABP is readily available and technically easy to use. Although it is usually placed through a femoral arterial approach, it can also be placed percutaneously or surgically through an axillary or subclavian arterial approach and, rarely, through the

Table 3
Comparison of temporary MCS devices

	IABP	Impella	TandemHeart	VA-ECMO
Cardiac flow (L/min)	0.3–0.5	1-5 (Impella 2.5, Impella CP, Impella 5)	2.5–5.0	3–7
Mechanism	AO	LV → AO	LA → AO	RA → AO
Maximum implant days	Weeks	7 d	14 d	Weeks
Sheath size	7–8 Fr	13–14 Fr Impella 5.0–21 Fr	15–17 Fr arterial; 21 Fr venous	14–16 Fr arterial; 18–21 Fr venous
Femoral artery size	>4 mm	Impella 2.5 and CP: 5–5.5 mm; Impella: 5–8 mm	8 mm	8 mm
Cardiac synchrony or stable rhythm	Yes	No	No	No
Afterload	↓	↓	↑	↑↑↑

MAP	↑	↑↑	↑↑
Cardiac flow	↑	↑↑	↑↑
Cardiac power	↑	↑↑	↑↑
LVEDP	↓	↓↓	↔
PCWP	↓	↓↓	↔
LV preload	—	↓↓	↓
Coronary perfusion	↑	↑	—
Myocardial oxygen demand	↓	↔↓	↔

Abbreviations: AO, aorta; IABP, intraaortic balloon pump; LV, left ventricle; LVEDP, left ventricular end-diastolic pressure; MAP, mean arterial pressure; RA, right atrium; VA-ECMO, venoarterial extracorporeal membrane oxygenation.

From Atkinson TM, Ohman EM, O'Neill WW, et al. A practical approach to mechanical circulatory support in patients undergoing percutaneous coronary intervention: an interventional perspective. JACC Cardiovasc Interv 2016;9(9):874; with permission.

brachial artery. Complications include local vascular injury, including bleeding and limb ischemia, as well as infection, thrombocytopenia, and rarely bowel or renal ischemia. It is contraindicated in patients with severe peripheral vascular disease, moderate to severe aortic regurgitation, and aortic disease.[15]

The IABP was shown to have benefit in earlier observational studies in patients with acute myocardial infarction and cardiogenic shock who were treated with fibrinolytic therapy. However, subsequent studies (CRISP-AMI trial) did not show any survival benefit.[16] The Shock II trial showed no differences in 30-day or 1-year mortality between those with and without IABP support.[17] The BCIS-1 study in high-risk patients undergoing percutaneous coronary intervention also failed to show a survival benefit, although the patients who had an IABP placed had less periprocedural hypotension.[18] Recently, a large randomized controlled trial (ISAR-SHOCK II) did not show any additional benefit of placing an IABP in patients with acute myocardial infarction and cardiogenic shock.

The use of IABP support remains a class 2 indication and is particularly recommended for those patients with cardiogenic shock who have an associated mechanical complication of mitral regurgitation or a ventricular septal defect.[19–22] It is also recommended when other forms of mechanical circulatory support are contraindicated or unavailable. It can be used with VA-ECMO.

The Impella 2.5 and the Impella CP

The Impella 2.5 and CP (Abiomed Inc) devices are microaxial pump devices placed percutaneously, most commonly through a femoral arterial approach and advanced in retrograde fashion across the aortic valve into the left ventricle. These devices help in direct unloading of the left ventricle and provide 1 to 4 L/min of flow. They increase the CPO and coronary perfusion. Newer percutaneous techniques to place these devices through an axillary arterial approach have been reported. The use of the Impella has been steadily increasing over the last few years owing to increased availability, user familiarity, and relative ease of deployment. However, they remain very expensive. It can be used along with VA-ECMO. Complications include device thrombosis, local vascular injury, limb ischemia, hemolysis, and infection. It is contraindicated in patients with LV thrombus, mechanical aortic valve, moderate to severe aortic regurgitation, and severe peripheral vascular disease.

Small randomized controlled trials (PROTECT I and PROTECT II) in patients undergoing high-risk percutaneous coronary intervention and the ISAR-SHOCK trial in patients with cardiogenic shock did not show a survival benefit, although the Impella 2.5 was shown to provide better hemodynamic support with a greater improvement in cardiac index. Registry data (EuroPella and USPella) have also shown better hemodynamic support with improved survival to discharge.[23–26]

TandemHeart

The TandemHeart (CardiacAssist Inc) is a continuous flow centrifugal device that bypasses the left ventricle. It helps in drawing blood from the left atrium (through a transseptally placed cannula) and pumps (uses a centrifugal pump 3500–7000 rpm) the blood back into the femoral/iliac arteries through an arterial cannula (left atrium–femoral artery pump). It provides 3 to 5 L/min of flow (depending on the size of the arterial cannula) and significantly decreases the LV preload. It can increase afterload and rarely an IABP can be used with it. It increases cardiac power output (CPO).[12]

It is contraindicated in patients with severe peripheral vascular disease, moderate to severe aortic regurgitation, ventricular septal defect, bleeding diathesis, and left atrial thrombus. Complications include local vascular injury, limb ischemia, air embolism, and thromboembolism. Rarely, the left atrial cannula can migrate into the right atrium, causing hemodynamic collapse and profound hypoxia. Small studies have shown that the TandemHeart provides superior hemodynamic support; however, this finding is not associated with survival benefit.[27]

Venoarterial extracorporeal membrane oxygenation

Peripherally inserted venoarterial extracorporeal membrane oxygenation device by-passes both the right and left side of the heart. It draws blood from the right atrium or central vein (venous cannula) and delivers oxygenated blood into femoral/iliac arteries. It is an ideal device for patients in refractory shock with hypoxia and with biventricular failure. It is relatively easy to place and can be inserted without fluoroscopy making it an ideal device to salvage patients receiving active cardiopulmonary resuscitation. CardioHelp (Maquet, Rastatt, Germany) is a portable ECMO device helpful in transportation. It increases the mean arterial pressure and CPO. However, it does significantly increase afterload and myocardial oxygen demand. Also, it can cause LV distension that can result in irreversible myocardial damage if not promptly recognized and addressed (either by decreasing the afterload with IABP or direct unloading with an Impella or placement of surgical/percutaneous direct LV vent).

Complications include local vascular injury, bleeding, limb ischemia, air embolism, infection, and thrombosis. Rarely, it can cause upper torso hypoxia (Harlequin syndrome). It is contraindicated in severe peripheral vascular disease, patients with active bleeding, moderate to severe aortic regurgitation, and those that cannot be anticoagulated. Extracorporeal life-support organization Registry data have shown better hemodynamic support; however, no survival benefit has been shown.[28]

Investigational devices

Percutaneous Heart Pump (Thoratec, Abbott, Alameda, CA) is a percutaneous trans-valvular microaxial pump device that has a self-expandable sheath that expands to 24-Fr across the aortic valve. It is inserted through the femoral arterial approach and can give hemodynamic support of up to 5.0 L/min.

Aortix (Procyrion, Houston, TX) and Reitan pump (Cardiobridge, Hechingen, Germany) devices are deployed in the descending aorta similar to an IABP.[12]

Temporary Percutaneous Right Ventricular Mechanical Support Devices

For patients who have biventricular failure or isolated severe RV failure and cardiogenic shock, percutaneous RV mechanical support may be necessary. The devices available are listed in **Box 2**.[1] An algorithm for management of acute right ventricular failure in cardiogenic shock is described in **Fig. 3**.

Right Ventricular TandemHeart

The TandemHeart can be used to support the RV by pumping blood into the pulmonary artery either using a Protek-Duo catheter (CardiacAssist Inc) that has proximal inlet in the right atrium and distal outlet in the main pulmonary artery or placing 2 different catheters (one in the right atrium and other in the pulmonary artery). Complications include thrombosis, embolism, and bleeding.

Right Ventricular Impella or R-Pella

The R-Pella device was approved recently for commercial use in acute severe RV failure. It has a proximal inlet at the level of the inferior vena cava and the outlet in the

---

Box 2
Classification of temporary mechanical circulatory support of the right ventricle

A. Direct RV bypass:
  1. Axial Flow
     • Impella RP
  2. Centrifugal Flow
     • Tandem RVAD
     • Tandem Protek Duo

B. Indirect RV bypass:
  1. Centrifugal Flow
     • VA ECMO

Abbreviations: RV, right ventricle; RVAD, right ventricular assist device; VA ECMO, veno-arterial extracorporeal membrane oxygenator.

---

pulmonary artery. Complications include thrombosis, bleeding, and infection. The RECOVER-RP trial showed its safety and efficacy in providing hemodynamic support.[29]

Venoarterial extracorporeal membrane oxygenation
The venoarterial extracorporeal membrane oxygenation helps in unloading the RV and can support patients in acute RV failure, especially those with acute massive pulmonary embolism and cardiogenic shock.

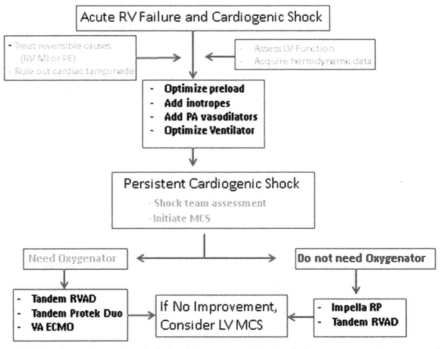

Fig. 3. Algorithm for mechanical circulatory support in RV failure. ECMO, extra-corporeal membrane oxygenator; LV, left ventricle; MCS, mechanical circulatory support; MI, myocardial infarction; PA, pulmonary artery; PE, pulmonary embolism; RV, right ventricle; RVAD, right ventricular assist device.

Future, prospective, randomized controlled trials are needed to evaluate if any of the devices available for temporary RV mechanical support improve survival in patients with RV failure and cardiogenic shock.

Surgical Temporary Mechanical Circulatory Support

Surgical implantation of a temporary mechanical circulatory support device requires a median sternotomy. The commercially available devices include the CentriMag device (Abbott), and Abiomed device (Abiomed Inc).

CentriMag
This device can be implanted surgically via a median sternotomy and used either in a univentricular or in a biventricular configuration. It is a centrifugal pump with a magnetically levitated rotor that can deliver flows up to 10 L/min. The inflow cannula is placed in the left atrium or in the LV apex and the outflow cannula in the ascending aorta. When used to support the right ventricle, the inflow cannula is placed in the right atrium and the outflow cannula in the pulmonary artery. There are no randomized controlled trials evaluating the survival benefit of this device.[1]

Abiomed AB 5000, Impella 5.0, and Impella LD
Similar to the CentriMag device, Abiomed AB5000 (Abiomed Inc, Danvers, MA) device can also be used in both a univentricular and biventricular configuration. This is a pulsatile pump that can generate flows of up to 6 L/min. No randomized controlled trials have been conducted with this device and there is no proven survival benefit with its use in cardiogenic shock.[1] This device has not been in use clinically recently. The Impella 5.0 and Impella LD (Abiomed Inc, Danvers, MA) are LV assist axial flow pump devices that need surgical placement and can provide up to 5.0 L/min of cardiac output.

Durable Mechanical Circulatory Support

Patients with cardiogenic shock who have been stabilized on medical therapy or on temporary mechanical circulatory support can be considered for durable mechanical circulatory support if they are suitable candidates. Current commercially available devices are all continuous flow devices and include the HeartMate 2 (Thoratec, Pleasanton, CA) axial flow pump, Heartware centrifugal flow pump (Heartware, Framingham, MA), and the HeartMate 3 centrifugal flow pump. All of these devices have been shown to improve both quality of life and survival in randomized controlled trials. These devices can be used either as a bridge to transplantation or recovery or as destination therapy. The use of these devices in hemodynamically unstable patients who remain in shock on temporary mechanical circulatory support therapy is not recommended because the surgical mortality is prohibitively high.[1]

SUMMARY

Cardiogenic shock continues to increase in prevalence and, despite progress in developing mechanical circulatory support options, the in-hospital mortality remains high. Myocardial dysfunction from acute coronary syndrome is the leading cause of cardiogenic shock. Early diagnosis, timely transfer to a tertiary or quaternary facility, and engagement of a multidisciplinary team that includes an interventional cardiologists, heart failure cardiologist, critical care medicine physician, and cardiac surgeon is necessary to achieve optimal clinical outcomes. Coronary revascularization must be considered in patients with acute coronary syndrome and evidence clearly demonstrates improved survival. In those patients who are not candidates for coronary revascularization, aggressive hemodynamically guided medical management and use of temporary percutaneous or surgical mechanical circulatory support is recommended. After hemodynamic stabilization is achieved, durable mechanical support may be an option in some patients.

REFERENCES

1. Van Diepen S, Katz JN, Albert NM, et al. Contemporary management of cardiogenic shock; a scientific statement from the American Heart Association. Circulation 2017;136(16):e232–68.
2. Sleeper LA, Reynolds HR, White HD, et al. A severity scoring system for risk assessment of patients with cardiogenic shock: a report from the SHOCK trial and registry. Am Heart J 2010;160:443–50.
3. Fuernau G, Thiele H. Intra-aortic balloon pump (IABP) in cardiogenic shock. Curr Opin Crit Care 2013;19(5):404–9.
4. Sandhu A, McCoy LA, Negi SI, et al. Use of mechanical circulatory support in patients undergoing percutaneous coronary intervention: insights from the National Cardiovascular Data Registry. Circulation 2015;132(13):1243–51.
5. Knaus WA, Draper EA, Wagner DP, et al. APACHE II: a severity of disease classification system. Crit Care Med 1985;13:818–29.
6. Knaus WA, Wagner DP, Draper EA, et al. The APACHE III prognostic system: risk prediction of hospital mortality for critically ill hospitalized adults. Chest 1991;100: 1619–36.
7. Le Gall JR, Lemeshow S, Saulnier F. A new simplified acute physiology score (SAPS II) based on a European/North American multicenter study. JAMA 1993; 270:2957–63 [Erratum appears in JAMA 1994;271:1321].
8. Harjola VP, Lassus J, Sionis A, et al. Clinical picture and risk prediction of short-term mortality in cardiogenic shock. Eur J Heart Fail 2015;17:501–9.
9. Thiele H, Akin I, Sandri M, et al. PCI strategies in patients with acute myocardial infarction and cardiogenic shock. N Engl J Med 2017;377:2419–32.
10. Atkinson TM, Ohman EM, O'Neill WW, et al. A practical approach to mechanical circulatory support in patients undergoing percutaneous coronary intervention: an interventional perspective. JACC Cardiovasc Interv 2016;9(9):871–83.
11. Jeger RV, Harkness SM, Ramanathan K, et al, SHOCK Investigators. Emergency revascularization in patients with cardiogenic shock on admission: a report from the SHOCK trial and registry. Eur Heart J 2006;27:664–70.
12. Burkhoff D, Sayer G, Doshi D, et al. Hemodynamics of mechanical circulatory support. J Am Coll Cardiol 2015;66(23):2663–74.
13. Fincke R, Hochman JS, Lowe AM, et al. Cardiac power is the strongest hemodynamic correlate of mortality in cardiogenic shock: a report from the SHOCK trial registry. J Am Coll Cardiol 2004;44(2):340–8.
14. Kantrowitz A, Tjonneland S, Freed PS, et al. Initial clinical experience with intra-aortic balloon pumping in cardiogenic shock. JAMA 1968;203(2):113–8.
15. Waksman R, Weiss AT, Gotsman MS, et al. Intra-aortic balloon counterpulsation improves survival in cardiogenic shock complicating acute myocardial infarction. Eur Heart J 1993;14(1):71–4.
16. Patel MR, Smalling RW, Thiele H, et al. Intra-aortic balloon counterpulsation and infarct size in patients with acute anterior myocardial infarction without shock: the CRISP AMI randomized trial. JAMA 2011;306(12):1329–37.
17. Thiele H, Zeymer U, Neumann FJ, et al. Intraaortic balloon support for myocardial infarction with cardiogenic shock. N Engl J Med 2012;367(14):1287–96.

18. Perera D, Stables R, Clayton T, et al, BCIS-1 Investigators. Long-term mortality data from the balloon pump-assisted coronary intervention study (BCIS-1): a randomized, controlled trial of elective balloon counterpulsation during high-risk percutaneous coronary intervention. Circulation 2013;127(2):207–12.
19. Hochman JS, Sleeper LA, Webb JG, et al. Early revascularization in acute myocardial infarction complicated by cardiogenic shock. SHOCK Investigators. Should we emergently revascularize occluded coronaries for cardiogenic shock. N Engl J Med 1999;341(9):625–34.
20. Perera D, Stables R, Thomas M, et al. Elective intra-aortic balloon counterpulsation during high-risk percutaneous coronary intervention: a randomized controlled trial. JAMA 2010;304(8):867–74.
21. Barron HV, Every NR, Parsons LS, et al. The use of intra-aortic balloon counterpulsation in patients with cardiogenic shock complicating acute myocardial infarction: data from the National Registry of Myocardial Infarction. Am Heart J 2001; 141(6):933–9.
22. Curtis JP, Rathore SS, Wang Y, et al. Use and effectiveness of intra-aortic balloon pumps among patients undergoing high risk percutaneous coronary intervention: insights from the National Cardiovascular Data Registry. Circ Cardiovasc Qual Outcomes 2012;5(1):21–30.
23. Dixon SR, Henriques JP, Mauri L, et al. A prospective feasibility trial investigating the use of the Impella 2.5 system in patients undergoing high-risk percutaneous coronary intervention (The PROTECT I Trial): initial U.S. experience. JACC Cardiovasc Interv 2009;2(2):91–6.
24. Maini B, Naidu SS, Mulukutla S, et al. Real-world use of the Impella 2.5 circulatory support system in complex high-risk percutaneous coronary intervention: the US-pella registry. Catheter Cardiovasc Interv 2012;80(5):717–25.
25. O'Neill WW, Kleiman NS, Moses J, et al. A prospective, randomized clinical trial of hemodynamic support with Impella 2.5 versus intra-aortic balloon pump in patients undergoing high-risk percutaneous coronary intervention: the PROTECT II study. Circulation 2012;126(14):1717–27.
26. Sjauw KD, Konorza T, Erbel R, et al. Supported high-risk percutaneous coronary intervention with the Impella 2.5 device the Europella registry. J Am Coll Cardiol 2009;54(25):2430–4.
27. Seyfarth M, Sibbing D, Bauer I, et al. A randomized clinical trial to evaluate the safety and efficacy of a percutaneous left ventricular assist device versus intra-aortic balloon pumping for treatment of cardiogenic shock caused by myocardial infarction. J Am Coll Cardiol 2008;52(19):1584–8.
28. Ouweneel DM, Schotborgh JV, Limpens J, et al. Extracorporeal life support during cardiac arrest and cardiogenic shock: a systematic review and meta-analysis. Intensive Care Med 2016;42(12):1922–34.
29. Anderson MB, Goldstein J, Milano C, et al. Benefits of a novel percutaneous ventricular assist device for right heart failure: the prospective RECOVER RIGHT study of the Impella RP device. J Heart Lung Transplant 2015;34(12):1549–60.

Prevention and Treatment of Right Ventricular Failure During Left Ventricular Assist Device Therapy

Amresh Raina, MD*, Maria Patarroyo-Aponte, MD

KEYWORDS

- Left ventricular assist device • Right ventricular failure • Morbidity • Mortality
- Risk stratification • Treatment • Prevention

KEY POINTS

- Right ventricular failure is a frequently encountered clinical problem due to the increasing utilization of left ventricular assist devices (LVADs) for end-stage heart failure and expansion of the patient population eligible for LVAD therapy.
- The true incidence of right ventricular failure post-LVAD implantation has been challenging to define because of varying definitions in the literature and switch from pulsatile to continuous flow technology.
- Postoperative right ventricular failure may be predicted by preoperative clinical, hemodynamic, and imaging variables, which have been combined into a variety of risk prediction algorithms, although right ventricular failure may also develop due to unanticipated intraoperative and postoperative factors.
- Early recognition of right ventricular failure is critical because early institution of medical therapy for right heart failure and/or right ventricular mechanical circulatory support is associated with superior outcomes versus delayed treatment.
- Randomized clinical trial data are needed to support the use of specific medical and device therapy in patients with right ventricular failure post-LVAD implant.

INTRODUCTION

Left ventricular assist devices (LVAD) are used with increasing frequency in patients with heart failure with reduced ejection fraction (HFrEF) and advanced heart failure

Disclosures: Dr A. Raina reports consulting fees from St. Jude and Actelion, speaking fees from United Therapeutics, Bayer, and Actelion. Dr M. Patarroyo-Aponte has no relevant disclosures.
Cardiovascular Institute, Allegheny General Hospital, 320 East North Avenue, Pittsburgh, PA 15212-4772, USA
* Corresponding author. Pulmonary Hypertension Program, Section of Heart Failure/Transplant/MCS & Pulmonary Hypertension, Allegheny General Hospital, Temple University School of Medicine, 320 East North Avenue, Pittsburgh, PA 15212-4772.
E-mail address: amresh.raina@ahn.org

(HF) symptoms despite maximally tolerated medical therapy.[1] Improvements in device design with smaller continuous flow (CF) pumps have improved device durability, and newer centrifugal pumps hold the promise of reducing serious adverse events, such as pump thrombosis.[2,3] With the increasing utilization of CF LVAD therapy and expansion of the patient population potentially eligible for LVAD implantation, right ventricular (RV) failure after LVAD implantation is more commonly encountered in clinical practice. The true incidence of RV failure after LVAD implantation is difficult to firmly establish because of varying definitions of RV failure in single-center studies and the shift from utilization of pulsatile to CF devices. Thus, estimates of the incidence of RV failure vary widely over a range from 10% to 40%.[4-7]

Severe RV failure after LVAD implantation and particularly requirement with a right ventricular assist device (RVAD) is associated with a substantial increase in morbidity and mortality and less successful bridging to cardiac transplantation.[1,5,6,8,9] Given that more LVAD patients with RV failure will be encountered clinically and the substantial impact RV failure has on LVAD outcomes, an important ongoing focus will be on strategies to identify and ideally prevent RV failure. In those patients who do develop RV failure, developing a treatment paradigm to improve outcomes remains a focus of discussion and continued research. In turn, a thorough understanding of mechanisms that are involved in the development of RV failure is required in order to prevent and treat it. This article reviews the following:

- The physiology underlying the development of RV failure in LVAD patients
- Established RV failure risk prediction algorithms
- Intraoperative and postoperative measures to try to prevent RV failure
- Management of patients who develop RV failure despite preoperative risk stratification, medical optimization, and aggressive perioperative treatment

DEFINITION OF RIGHT VENTRICULAR FAILURE

RV failure after LVAD implantation has been challenging to consistently define in the literature because there have been a variety of definitions in different single-center studies and most RV failure has been defined in relation to the index hospitalization for LVAD implant. The most consistently used and updated definition from the INTERMACs database characterizes RV failure as mild, moderate, or severe/severe-acute predominantly based on signs of elevated central venous pressure (CVP) and duration of inotropic/vasodilator support, need for RVAD implant, or death from RV failure after LVAD implant.[1] However, there is increasing recognition of a subset of patients who survive the index LVAD hospitalization without meeting criteria for severe RV failure but who subsequently present much later in their clinical course with symptomatic RV failure. These patients with "late" RV failure also have substantially increased morbidity and mortality.[10,11]

MECHANISMS OF RIGHT VENTRICULAR FAILURE

The development of RV failure can occur for a variety of reasons: some secondary to patient-related factors evident before LVAD implantation, others due to factors occurring during the intraoperative or perioperative course and additional issues that develop in the immediate postoperative period.

Preoperative Risk Factors

One of the biggest risk factors for postoperative RV failure is preoperative RV dysfunction. Biventricular dysfunction is common in patients with end-stage HFrEF of both ischemic and nonischemic causes and can occur due to the development of chronic secondary pulmonary hypertension (PH), left-sided valvular heart disease, particularly mitral regurgitation (MR), but also due to extension of the primary myopathic process that affects the left ventricle (LV) to the RV.[12–16]

Several parameters have been used to describe RV function (**Table 1**). RV dysfunction was initially defined by invasive hemodynamic parameters from preoperative right heart catheterization. Low RV stroke work index, defined as (mean pulmonary artery pressure [PA] – right atrial pressure/stroke volume index) is one such metric that has been associated with RV failure after LVAD implantation in single-center studies.[5,17] An even simpler hemodynamic measurement that can be calculated at bedside is CVP to pulmonary capillary wedge pressure (PCWP) ratio, with a ratio greater than 0.63 associated with development of postoperative RV failure.[6] Finally, a recent study in 132 CF LVADs suggested pulmonary arterial pulsatility index (PA systolic–PA diastolic/CVP) was additional hemodynamic metric superior to CVP:PCWP ratio, RV stroke work index, or CVP alone in predicting RV failure.[18]

Beyond invasive hemodynamic parameters, there has been increasing interest in echocardiographic assessment of preoperative RV function in prediction of postoperative RV failure. A variety of echocardiographic parameters have been associated with RV failure, predominantly derived again from relatively small single-center studies. For example, Puwanant and colleagues[19] demonstrated that tricuspid annular plane systolic excursion (TAPSE) at a cutoff of 8 mm was highly sensitive for predicting postoperative RV failure in a single-center study of mixed pulsatile and CF LVADs. Subsequently, a variety of additional echocardiographic measures of RV function, such as qualitative assessment of severe RV dysfunction, RV global free wall strain, and right ventricular fractional area change (RVFAC), have all been associated with post-LVAD RV failure in relatively small single-center studies.[5,20–22]

In addition to measurements of RV function, anatomic measurements of the right atrium, RV, and LV have been associated with RV failure. RV/LV ratio on intraoperative transesophageal echocardiogram or preoperative transthoracic echocardiogram, left atrial diameter to LV end-diastolic dimension, and left atrial volume index have also been associated with RV failure.[22–25] Finally, severe tricuspid valve regurgitation is another indirect echocardiographic surrogate of RV function that has been associated with RV failure post-LVAD implant.[20,26]

Table 1 Assessment of right ventricular function	
Echocardiography	• Qualitative assessment • Right atrium and RV size • RV/LV ratio • Left atrium volume index • TAPSE • RVFAC • RV global free wall strain • Tricuspid regurgitation severity
Hemodynamics	• RA/PCWP ratio • PA pulsatility index • RV stroke work index

However, preoperative RV dysfunction is clearly not the only explanation for the development of RV failure after LVAD implant. Indeed, in many patients with preoperative RV dysfunction before LVAD implantation, RV function can improve post-LVAD implant because of the decongestion of the LV, lowering of left heart–filling pressures, and decrease in secondary PH and tricuspid regurgitation.[27] Therefore, beyond the assessment of preoperative RV dysfunction using hemodynamics or echocardiographic variables, additional preoperative laboratory, demographic, and clinical variables have been evaluated in RV failure risk prediction scores.

Predicting Right Ventricular Failure: Risk Scores

Using multivariate analysis, a variety of preoperative variables have been combined into RV failure risk prediction scores. Unfortunately, many of these algorithms were developed in the era of pulsatile flow LVADs, have used varying definitions of RV failure, have predominantly been derived from single-center studies without large validation cohorts, and have had modest predictive value.[4–6,20,26,28]

The Michigan RV failure risk score was perhaps the first of these algorithms to be developed and incorporated preoperative variables, including vasopressor requirement, renal dysfunction, elevated bilirubin, and aspartate aminotransferase levels. In this cohort, most patients had pulsatile flow LVADs. Area under the curve (AUC) for this risk score was 0.73.[28] Fitzpatrick and colleagues[5] studied a cohort of 167 patients with predominantly pulsatile flow LVADs and developed a score that predicted the need for biventricular mechanical circulatory support. Components to the score included preoperative cardiac index, RV stroke work index, severe RV dysfunction by qualitative assessment on echocardiogram, preoperative creatinine, and previous cardiac surgery. Another study by Drakos and colleagues[4] studied 175 patients again with predominantly pulsatile LVADs and showed that preoperative intra-aortic balloon pump, inotrope dependency destination therapy LVAD indication, β-blocker use, ACE inhibitor use, elevated pulmonary vascular resistance (PVR), and obesity were associated with RV failure. AUC for this score was similar to the Michigan score at 0.74.

In the more contemporary CF LVAD era, Kormos and colleagues[6] developed a preoperative score using the HeartMate II bridge to transplant data and found that CVP:PCWP ratio greater than 0.63, need for preoperative ventilatory support, or elevated blood urea nitrogen (BUN) greater than 39 mg/dL were associated with RV failure. Kato and colleagues[23] evaluated 111 patients with predominantly CF devices and found that LV diastolic dimension, left ventricular ejection fraction, left atrial diameter divided by LV diastolic dimension, bilirubin, and RV stroke work index were associated with RV failure with an AUC of 0.789. Atluri and colleagues[20] evaluated a contemporary cohort of 218 CF LVADs and found the elevated CVP greater than 15 mm Hg, qualitative severe RV dysfunction, preoperative intubation, severe tricuspid regurgitation, and preoperative tachycardia were associated with RV failure. Vivo and colleagues[25] and Kukucka and colleagues[24] evaluated a relatively simple echocardiographic metric of RV-to-LV end-diastolic ratio from either transthoracic echocardiogram or transesophageal echocardiogram at the time of LVAD implant with similar AUC of 0.68 and 0.74 to the more complex scores. Aissaoui and colleagues[29] combined several echocardiographic metrics, including RVFAC, basal RV end-diastolic diameter, RV tissue Doppler systolic velocity, and TAPSE with INTERMACs implant classification and found that a score greater than 3 predicted the occurrence of right ventricular failure with 89% sensitivity and 74% specificity. Bellavia and colleagues[30] recently published a meta-analysis of observational studies evaluating RV failure after LVAD implant with overall incidence of 35%. In this study, the investigators reported that the principal risk factors associated with RV failure were clinical factors (need for mechanical ventilation, renal replacement therapy), biochemical markers (international normalized ratio and N-terminal prohormone of brain natriuretic peptide), hemodynamic measures (RV stroke work index and CVP), and echocardiographic measurements (preimplant moderate to severe RV dysfunction assessed qualitatively or a greater RV/LV diameter). Most recently, Kashiyama and colleagues[31] showed that addition of liver stiffness (a measure closely related to right-sided filling pressures) to other parameters can predict RV failure after LVAD with an AUC of 0.89.

Unfortunately, one of the problems with risk prediction scores is that they have not been well validated outside of their derivation cohorts, and their predictive value in validation cohorts is likely lower than in the derivation cohorts. Pettinari and colleagues[32] evaluated 3 of the previously published RV risk scores in a series of 59 LVAD implants and found that the risk scores were not significantly different in patients who needed temporary RV mechanical support versus those who did not. Kalogeropoulos and colleagues[33] evaluated 6 of the currently available RV failure risk prediction models and found that all of these algorithms performed modestly when applied to external populations outside their original derivation cohort. A more sophisticated approach to RV failure risk prediction may be using a Bayesian prognostic model that incorporates multiple preoperative risk factors as well as their interaction (**Table 2**). The AUC of the Bayesian model using data from the large INTERMACs registry was 0.90 for acute (<48 hours after implant) RV failure, 0.84 for early (48 hours to 14 days) RV failure, and 0.88 for late (>14 days) RV failure after LVAD implantation.[34]

Intraoperative and Perioperative Factors

In some patients, RV dysfunction can develop de novo after LVAD implantation, and in others, mild or moderate preoperative RV dysfunction can progress to frank RV failure due to factors that develop in the operating room or in the immediate perioperative period.

Durable LVAD implantation is still performed at most centers using full sternotomy and cardiopulmonary bypass. Cardioplegia can, despite myocardial protection, lead to relative stunning of the myocardium, particularly the RV, which is not directly unloaded by the LVAD postoperatively. In addition, cardiopulmonary bypass can cause cytokine release, systemic inflammatory response syndrome (SIRS), as well as elevations in PVR, which can stress an already dysfunctional RV.[35] Moreover, other intraoperative problems, such as myocardial ischemia, air embolism to the right coronary artery, mechanical compression of the PA, and tamponade, can all contribute to RV failure.[7]

LVAD circulatory physiology can also contribute to RV failure after implant. After LVAD implantation, there is increased flow from the LV/LVAD and increased venous return to the RV, resulting in an increase in RV preload. In addition, after LVAD

Table 2					
Performance of Bayesian risk score for predicting right ventricular failure after left ventricular assist device implantation					
Clinical Endpoint	**Accuracy (%)**	**AUC (%)**	**Sensitivity (%)**	**Specificity (%)**	**No. of Variables**
Acute RVF (<48 h)	97.3	90.3	80.0	99.7	33
Early RVF (>48 h to <14 d)	91.2	83.5	67.2	98.7	34
Late RVF (>14 d)	94.5	88.3	75.1	99.7	34

implantation, there is often loss of the septal contribution to overall RV function with postoperative paradoxic septal motion. In these patients, despite the objective decrease in ventricular afterload, the CVP remained unchanged and the ratio between CVP and PCWP worsened early after LVAD, suggesting poor RV adaptation early after LVAD with progressive improvement over time.[36] Finally, the increased venous return to the RV can in some instances, particularly with aggressive or rapid titration of LVAD speed, result in the interventricular septum being pulled toward LV, worsening right heart dimensions and tricuspid regurgitation.[25,27,36–38]

A variety of other perioperative or immediate postoperative factors can contribute to right HF. Acute hypoxemia perioperatively can result in pulmonary vasoconstriction, worsening PVR, and associated RV dysfunction. Acute renal dysfunction with secondary increase in CVP as well as metabolic and/or respiratory acidosis can contribute to a lack of vasopressor responsiveness.[39] Redo sternotomy with increased risk of perioperative bleeding and transfusion requirement has been associated with SIRS and worsening RV function. Sustained atrial and in particular ventricular tachyarrhythmias can also worsen RV function.[40]

PREVENTION OF RIGHT VENTRICULAR FAILURE
Preoperative Optimization

Other than patient selection and identification of patients at risk for RV failure using some of the risk stratification tools detailed above, preoperative optimization in patients who present with decompensated HF is imperative to prevent postoperative RV failure. The essential principles of preoperative management include optimization of preload, afterload, and contractility. Typically, diuretics should be used to maintain CVP less than 15 mm Hg if feasible. Inotropes such as milrinone or dobutamine should be used cautiously to optimize cardiac index and hemodynamics before LVAD implantation. These agents also have vasodilatory affects and so may improve systemic vascular resistance and to a lesser extent PVR. In patients who remain hemodynamically compromised, temporary mechanical support devices, such as an intra-aortic balloon pump (although associated with RV failure in some studies) or other percutaneous devices, such as Impella, may be used to optimize end-organ function. Correction of coagulopathy is also important in terms of minimizing postoperative bleeding and transfusion requirement. In patients with critical cardiogenic shock and INTERMACS 1 clinical profile, consideration should be made of bridging with temporary mechanical circulatory support or venoarterial extracorporeal membrane oxygenation (ECMO) to stabilize hemodynamics end-organ function before consideration of durable LVAD.

Intraoperative Optimization

As detailed above, a variety of intraoperative factors may result in worsening right heart function. Surgical technique with limitation of cardiopulmonary bypass time and careful myocardial preservation can help to diminish risk of RV stunning with cardiopulmonary bypass. Careful attention to bleeding can limit the requirement for transfusion, which may prevent SIRS and transfusion-related lung injury. Meticulous attention to proper deairing could also help to avoid air embolism to the right coronary artery. With close attention to acid-base balance and ventilatory status, acidosis can be avoided as can hypoxemia and hypercapnia. Delayed sternal closure can also be used in LVAD patients, particularly patients with previous cardiac surgery and coagulopathy, and this may ameliorate risk of cardiac tamponade and mechanical compression of the RV and PA.

In the operating room, a decision must often be made with regards to repair of the tricuspid valve because tricuspid regurgitation can worsen after LVAD implant because of leftward interventricular septal shift.[41] Moreover, severe tricuspid regurgitation has been associated with the development of postoperative RV failure.[20,26] Some studies have suggested that tricuspid repair is associated with decreased risk of RV failure and improved morbidity/mortality. However, a large meta-analysis suggested no benefit of routine tricuspid valve repair in terms of reducing early mortality or need for RVAD in patients with moderate to severe tricuspid regurgitation.[42]

With regards to MR, in general, with LV decompression with the LVAD, MR decreases, and consequently, there has not been much impetus to repair or replace the mitral valve at the time of LVAD implantation. However, a recent study suggested that patients with residual MR after LVAD implantation had larger postoperative RV dimensions, worse postoperative RV function, and adverse clinical outcomes (**Table 3**).[43] A recent small observational study also showed that overall survival and freedom from recurrent MR were significantly better in patients who underwent surgical repair of MR at the time of LVAD.[44] Despite these data, the role of mitral repair remains controversial in LVAD patients, and literature on this topic is still developing.

Cautious optimization of LVAD speed is critically important in the operating room immediately postoperatively. Overly aggressive titration of LVAD speed can cause shift of the ventricular septum toward the LV, impacting RV performance, and can also potentially cause ventricular tachycardia via contact of the ventricular septum to the LVAD inflow cannula. In the operating room, LVAD speed should be cautiously titrated using transesophageal echocardiographic guidance to optimize aortic valve opening and septal position.[24,39]

Postoperative Measures

In the immediate postoperative period, typically patients should be carefully managed using hemodynamic guidance. Inotropes such as dobutamine or milrinone are typically used to optimize cardiac output and LVAD filling. In patients with relative hypotension, epinephrine and to a lesser extent norepinephrine are commonly used.

Avoiding hypoxemia and hypercapnia is critically important in the postoperative period. In patients with severe intraoperative or perioperative hypoxemic,

Table 3
Relationship of residual mitral regurgitation after left ventricular assist devices implant to right ventricular dysfunction and clinical outcomes

Parameter	Preoperative Data (n = 69)	Residual MR Cohort (n = 14)	No Residual MR Cohort (n = 55)	P Value
RVEDD (mm)	48 ± 8	49 ± 6	45 ± 9	.04
TAPSE (mm)	14 ± 4	10 ± 2	12 ± 3	.02
RVFAC (%)	26 ± 12	29 ± 5	34 ± 9	.02
Tricuspid regurgitation jet (mm Hg)	38 ± 13	26 ± 7	25 ± 10	.79
PA systolic pressure (mm Hg)	51 ± 14	35 ± 9	34 ± 11	.85
RVOT VTI (cm)	12 ± 4	13 ± 4	16 ± 12	.13
Time from LVAD implant to first hospitalization (d)	—	62 ± 34	103 ± 112	.05
Time from LVAD implant to death (d)	—	80 ± 11	421 ± 514	.03

Abbreviations: RVEDD, right ventricular end diastolic dimension; VTI, velocity time integral.

consideration of venovenous ECMO should be made. Maintaining adequate oxygenation and ventilation is also important after extubation, and supplementary oxygen and/or noninvasive positive-pressure ventilation may be used in these situations.

Inhaled nitric oxide has been frequently used in patients with preoperative PH and/or RV dysfunction. A prospective, randomized clinical trial of inhaled nitric oxide in 150 patients undergoing LVAD implant with elevated PVR did not suggest overall benefit in terms of prevention of RV failure or mortality, but there was a signal toward benefit in patients with elevated PA pressures and PVR.[45] Unfortunately, although inhaled vasodilatory agents have the potential to decrease pulmonary pressures in the postoperative period with low incidence of RVF and improvement in survival when used early, there is a still lack of large randomized clinical studies to support their use as well as guidance regarding doses and agent selection.[46] In this regard, Sabato and colleagues[47] propose that the medical treatment of RV failure should be based on the presence or absence of elevated PVR. Thus, if RV failure occurs in the setting of normal PVR, inotropic agents such as dobutamine should be used, but if the PVR is elevated (>3 Wood units) or the patient has a transpulmonary gradient higher than 12 mm Hg, then an inhaled pulmonary vasodilator agent should be considered.

TREATMENT OF RIGHT VENTRICULAR FAILURE
Available Medical Treatment Options for Right Ventricular Failure Are Categorized

Acute and early right ventricular failure
While treating RV failure, therapy should be directed toward the same physiologic principles as in prevention namely optimization of preload, afterload, and contractility (**Table 4**). Device parameters should be reviewed carefully to understand the interaction between the LVAD and the patient's heart, including LV dimensions, septal position, aortic valve opening, MR, pump speed, and assessment of RV function.

Table 4
Treatment of right ventricular failure

	Acute RV Failure (<48 h)	Early RV Failure (48 h to <14 d)	Late RV Failure (>14 d)
RV preload	Optimize volume status with diuresis, ultrafiltration, transfusion	Optimize volume status with diuresis, ultrafiltration	Optimize volume status with diuresis
RV afterload	Inhaled nitric oxide	Inhaled prostanoid or oral PDE5 inhibitors	Oral PDE5 inhibitors
RV contractility	Epinephrine	Dobutamine or milrinone	Digoxin
Arrhythmias	Manage atrial and ventricular arrhythmias	Manage atrial and ventricular arrhythmias	Manage atrial and ventricular arrhythmias
Mechanical support	V-A and/or V-V ECMO, TandemHeart, RP Impella	TandemHeart, RP Impella	
LVAD parameters		Optimize LVAD parameters	Optimize LVAD parameters with echocardiographic and/or invasive hemodynamic ramp study

Patients with RV failure will typically have right heart congestion with elevated CVP and elevated right heart preload, impacting septal position and LVAD filling. Therefore, RV failure results in low indices of LVAD pulsatility on waveform analysis or pulsatility index. In this situation, typically aggressive diuresis and potentially ultrafiltration are required for volume removal to achieve CVP less than 15 mm Hg. In terms of lowering RV afterload, pulmonary vasodilating therapy, typically with inhaled nitric oxide or inhaled prostacyclins, is commonly used if PA pressures and PVR are elevated. Alternatively, phosphodiesterase type 5 (PDE5) inhibitors such as sildenafil may be used in patients who are not profoundly hypotensive, although the evidence supporting their use in the treatment of these patients is weak and mostly based on small studies and retrospective cohorts.[45,48–50] In terms of optimizing contractility and cardiac output, inotropic therapy, typically with dobutamine or milrinone, is often needed to optimize end-organ perfusion as well as LVAD filling. Epinephrine, norepinephrine, and dopamine are sometimes used in patients who are hypotensive.[41]

In patients with severe acute RV failure, consideration of early use of a temporary mechanical support device should be made. Studies have shown that planned or early RVAD implantation is associated with superior outcomes versus delayed or rescue placement, specifically with addition of in-line ECMO, which decreases 30-day mortality compared with patients that underwent RVAD alone.[51–53] Fortunately, there are an increasing number of options for temporary RVAD support. Centrally cannulated devices include centrifugal pumps, such as the CentriMag (Abbott, St Paul, MN) or Revolution (Sorin, Arvada, CO). However, there are now additional percutaneous RV support devices that are available, such as RV tandem heart (CardiacAssist, Pittsburgh, PA) or RP Impella (Abiomed, Danvers, MA) percutaneous devices.[54,55] The goal of temporary mechanical support placement is to support the failing RV and preserve LVAD filling and end-organ perfusion in the hopes that there will be gradual and consistent improvement in RV function, which will allow weaning of the RV support device, although in some patients use of temporary RVAD for more than 7 days with blood flow greater than 4 L/min has been associated with pulmonary hemorrhage.[56] In some patients, however, RV failure is persistent and consideration of a durable RVAD can be made in patients who are not likely to be emergently transplanted. In this situation, there have been numerous reports of utilization of a right-sided HeartWare CF device, cannulated either to the right atrium or to a portion of the RV and with outflow graft connected to the PA.[57,58]

Late right ventricular failure
The bulk of the established literature as detailed above has focused on the development of RV failure in the immediate postoperative period. However, there is much less known about the development of late RV failure, but this may be of increasing clinical importance. In some patients, late RV failure can develop secondary to inadequate unloading from the LVAD, which in turn can occur due to mechanical LVAD dysfunction, aortic or mitral regurgitant lesions, or inadequate blood pressure management. However, in other patients, primary RV dysfunction/RV failure occurs with normal LVAD function.

Again, there has been fairly little consensus with regards to what defines truly "late" RV failure. In a single-center study by Kapelios and colleagues,[10] at a median of 2.1 years after LVAD implant, 45% of patients developed signs or symptoms of right HF. In this study, there was no association between preoperative variables in those that developed late RV failure versus those who did not. A further 44% of the patients who developed late RV failure subsequently died during follow-up, illustrating the impact of late RV failure on outcomes. In another cohort studied by Takeda and

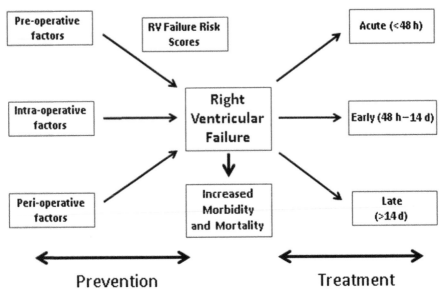

Fig. 1. RV failure in LVAD patients.

colleagues[11] with CF LVADs, 11% developed late right HF at a median of 99 days after discharge after LVAD implant. Several preimplant variables, including body mass index greater than 29, BUN greater than 41, and diabetes mellitus, were significant predictors of late right HF in this study. Of note, late RV failure during LVAD support has been also associated with worse 5-year posttransplant survival compared with patients who did not develop RV failure.[59]

In these patients, pump speed optimization after LVAD by echocardiographic and/or invasive hemodynamic RAMP study can lead to improvement in RVFAC and RV longitudinal peak systolic strain, suggesting that speed optimization in stable LVAD patients can improve RV function.

SUMMARY

Although CF LVADs offer the promise of smaller and more reliable devices designed for long-term hemodynamic support, RV failure is still a problem in more than one-third of patients early after LVAD implant (**Fig. 1**). RV failure either early or late after LVAD implant is associated with a substantial increase in morbidity and mortality, even for LVAD patients who are candidates for cardiac transplantation. Prevention of RV failure may be achieved through careful patient selection, through use of preoperative risk prediction tools to identify more appropriate LVAD candidates, and by careful preoperative optimization and perioperative management. Early recognition of RV failure is key to improving outcomes in these patients independent of the therapy used (either medical therapy or mechanical circulatory support or both). There is nonetheless a need for large, randomized studies to evaluate the currently available therapies for RV failure, including inhaled vasodilatory agents and temporary mechanical support.

REFERENCES

1. Kirklin JK, Pagani FD, Kormos RL, et al. Eighth annual INTERMACS report: special focus on framing the impact of adverse events. J Heart Lung Transplant 2017;36(10):1080–6.

2. Mehra MR, Naka Y, Uriel N, et al. A fully magnetically levitated circulatory pump for advanced heart failure. N Engl J Med 2017;376(5):440–50.

3. Rogers JG, Pagani FD, Tatooles AJ, et al. Intrapericardial left ventricular assist device for advanced heart failure. N Engl J Med 2017;376(5):451–60.

4. Drakos SG, Janicki L, Horne BD, et al. Risk factors predictive of right ventricular failure after left ventricular assist device implantation. Am J Cardiol 2010;105(7): 1030–5.

5. Fitzpatrick JR 3rd, Frederick JR, Hsu VM, et al. Risk score derived from preoperative data analysis predicts the need for biventricular mechanical circulatory support. J Heart Lung Transpl 2008;27(12):1286–92.

6. Kormos RL, Teuteberg JJ, Pagani FD, et al. Right ventricular failure in patients with the HeartMate II continuous-flow left ventricular assist device: incidence, risk factors, and effect on outcomes. J Thorac Cardiovasc Surg 2010;139(5): 1316–24.

7. Patlolla B, Beygui R, Haddad F. Right-ventricular failure following left ventricle assist device implantation. Curr Opin Cardiol 2013;28(2):223–33.

8. LaRue SJ, Raymer DS, Pierce BR, et al. Clinical outcomes associated with INTERMACS-defined right heart failure after left ventricular assist device implantation. J Heart Lung Transpl 2017;36(4):475–7.

9. Takeda K, Naka Y, Yang JA, et al. Outcome of unplanned right ventricular assist device support for severe right heart failure after implantable left ventricular assist device insertion. J Heart Lung Transpl 2014;33(2):141–8.

10. Kapelios CJ, Charitos C, Kaldara E, et al. Late-onset right ventricular dysfunction after mechanical support by a continuous-flow left ventricular assist device. J Heart Lung Transpl 2015;34(12):1604–10.

11. Takeda K, Takayama H, Colombo PC, et al. Incidence and clinical significance of late right heart failure during continuous-flow left ventricular assist device support. J Heart Lung Transpl 2015;34(8):1024–32.

12. Bosch L, Lam CSP, Gong L, et al. Right ventricular dysfunction in left-sided heart failure with preserved versus reduced ejection fraction. Eur J Heart Fail 2017; 19(12):1664–71.

13. Ghio S, Guazzi M, Scardovi AB, et al. Different correlates but similar prognostic implications for right ventricular dysfunction in heart failure patients with reduced or preserved ejection fraction. Eur J Heart Fail 2017;19(7):873–9.

14. Guazzi M, Naeije R. Pulmonary hypertension in heart failure: pathophysiology, pathobiology, and emerging clinical perspectives. J Am Coll Cardiol 2017; 69(13):1718–34.

15. Pfisterer M, Emmenegger H, Muller-Brand J, et al. Prevalence and extent of right ventricular dysfunction after myocardial infarction–relation to location and extent of infarction and left ventricular function. Int J Cardiol 1990;28(3):325–32.

16. Pueschner A, Chattranukulchai P, Heitner JF, et al. The prevalence, correlates, and impact on cardiac mortality of right ventricular dysfunction in nonischemic cardiomyopathy. JACC Cardiovasc Imaging 2017;10(10 Pt B):1225–36.

17. Ochiai Y, McCarthy PM, Smedira NG, et al. Predictors of severe right ventricular failure after implantable left ventricular assist device insertion: analysis of 245 patients. Circulation 2002;106(12 suppl 1):I198–202.

18. Morine KJ, Kiernan MS, Pham DT, et al. Pulmonary artery pulsatility index is associated with right ventricular failure after left ventricular assist device surgery. J Card Fail 2016;22(2):110–6.

19. Puwanant S, Hamilton KK, Klodell CT, et al. Tricuspid annular motion as a predictor of severe right ventricular failure after left ventricular assist device implantation. J Heart Lung Transpl 2008;27(10):1102–7.
20. Atluri P, Goldstone AB, Fairman AS, et al. Predicting right ventricular failure in the modern, continuous flow left ventricular assist device era. Ann Thorac Surg 2013; 96(3):857–63 [discussion: 63–64].
21. Grant AD, Smedira NG, Starling RC, et al. Independent and incremental role of quantitative right ventricular evaluation for the prediction of right ventricular failure after left ventricular assist device implantation. J Am Coll Cardiol 2012;60(6): 521–8.
22. Raina A, Seetha Rammohan HR, Gertz ZM, et al. Postoperative right ventricular failure after left ventricular assist device placement is predicted by preoperative echocardiographic structural, hemodynamic, and functional parameters. J Card Fail 2013;19(1):16–24.
23. Kato TS, Farr M, Schulze PC, et al. Usefulness of two-dimensional echocardiographic parameters of the left side of the heart to predict right ventricular failure after left ventricular assist device implantation. Am J Cardiol 2012;109(2):246–51.
24. Kukucka M, Stepanenko A, Potapov E, et al. Right-to-left ventricular end-diastolic diameter ratio and prediction of right ventricular failure with continuous-flow left ventricular assist devices. J Heart Lung Transpl 2011;30(1):64–9.
25. Vivo RP, Cordero-Reyes AM, Qamar U, et al. Increased right-to-left ventricle diameter ratio is a strong predictor of right ventricular failure after left ventricular assist device. J Heart Lung Transpl 2013;32(8):792–9.
26. Potapov EV, Stepanenko A, Dandel M, et al. Tricuspid incompetence and geometry of the right ventricle as predictors of right ventricular function after implantation of a left ventricular assist device. J Heart Lung Transpl 2008;27(12):1275–81.
27. Atluri P, Fairman AS, MacArthur JW, et al. Continuous flow left ventricular assist device implant significantly improves pulmonary hypertension, right ventricular contractility, and tricuspid valve competence. J Card Surg 2013;28(6):770–5.
28. Matthews JC, Koelling TM, Pagani FD, et al. The right ventricular failure risk score a pre-operative tool for assessing the risk of right ventricular failure in left ventricular assist device candidates. J Am Coll Cardiol 2008;51(22):2163–72.
29. Aissaoui N, Salem JE, Paluszkiewicz L, et al. Assessment of right ventricular dysfunction predictors before the implantation of a left ventricular assist device in end-stage heart failure patients using echocardiographic measures (ARVADE): combination of left and right ventricular echocardiographic variables. Arch Cardiovasc Dis 2015;108(5):300–9.
30. Bellavia D, Iacovoni A, Scardulla C, et al. Prediction of right ventricular failure after ventricular assist device implant: systematic review and meta-analysis of observational studies. Eur J Heart Fail 2017;19(7):926–46.
31. Kashiyama N, Toda K, Nakamura T, et al. Evaluation of right ventricular function using liver stiffness in patients with left ventricular assist device. Eur J Cardiothorac Surg 2017;51(4):715–21.
32. Pettinari M, Jacobs S, Rega F, et al. Are right ventricular risk scores useful? Eur J Cardiothorac Surg 2012;42(4):621–6.
33. Kalogeropoulos AP, Kelkar A, Weinberger JF, et al. Validation of clinical scores for right ventricular failure prediction after implantation of continuous-flow left ventricular assist devices. J Heart Lung Transpl 2015;34(12):1595–603.
34. Loghmanpour NA, Kormos RL, Kanwar MK, et al. A Bayesian model to predict right ventricular failure following left ventricular assist device therapy. JACC Heart Fail 2016;4(9):711–21.

35. Denault AY, Couture P, Beaulieu Y, et al. Right ventricular depression after cardiopulmonary bypass for valvular surgery. J Cardiothorac Vasc Anesth 2015;29(4):836–44.
36. Houston BA, Kalathiya RJ, Hsu S, et al. Right ventricular afterload sensitivity dramatically increases after left ventricular assist device implantation: a multicenter hemodynamic analysis. J Heart Lung Transpl 2016;35(7):868–76.
37. Kiernan MS, French AL, DeNofrio D, et al. Preoperative three-dimensional echocardiography to assess risk of right ventricular failure after left ventricular assist device surgery. J Card Fail 2015;21(3):189–97.
38. Holman WL, Bourge RC, Fan P, et al. Influence of left ventricular assist on valvular regurgitation. Circulation 1993;88(5 Pt 2):II309–I318.
39. Meineri M, Van Rensburg AE, Vegas A. Right ventricular failure after LVAD implantation: prevention and treatment. Best Pract Res Clin Anaesthesiol 2012;26(2):217–29.
40. Lampert BC, Teuteberg JJ. Right ventricular failure after left ventricular assist devices. J Heart Lung Transpl 2015;34(9):1123–30.
41. Slaughter MS, Pagani FD, Rogers JG, et al. Clinical management of continuous-flow left ventricular assist devices in advanced heart failure. J Heart Lung Transpl 2010;29(4 suppl):S1–39.
42. Robertson JO, Grau-Sepulveda MV, Okada S, et al. Concomitant tricuspid valve surgery during implantation of continuous-flow left ventricular assist devices: a Society of Thoracic Surgeons database analysis. J Heart Lung Transpl 2014;33(6):609–17.
43. Kassis H, Cherukuri K, Agarwal R, et al. Significance of residual mitral regurgitation after continuous flow left ventricular assist device implantation. JACC Heart Fail 2017;5(2):81–8.
44. Tanaka A, Onsager D, Song T, et al. Surgically corrected mitral regurgitation during left ventricular assist device implantation is associated with low recurrence rate and improved midterm survival. Ann Thorac Surg 2017;103(3):725–33.
45. Potapov E, Meyer D, Swaminathan M, et al. Inhaled nitric oxide after left ventricular assist device implantation: a prospective, randomized, double-blind, multicenter, placebo-controlled trial. J Heart Lung Transpl 2011;30(8):870–8.
46. Critoph C, Green G, Hayes H, et al. Clinical outcomes of patients treated with pulmonary vasodilators early and in high dose after left ventricular assist device implantation. Artif Organs 2016;40(1):106–14.
47. Sabato LA, Salerno DM, Moretz JD, et al. Inhaled pulmonary vasodilator therapy for management of right ventricular dysfunction after left ventricular assist device placement and cardiac transplantation. Pharmacotherapy 2017;37(8):944–55.
48. Tedford RJ, Hemnes AR, Russell SD, et al. PDE5A inhibitor treatment of persistent pulmonary hypertension after mechanical circulatory support. Circ Heart Fail 2008;1(4):213–9.
49. Groves DS, Blum FE, Huffmyer JL, et al. Effects of early inhaled epoprostenol therapy on pulmonary artery pressure and blood loss during LVAD placement. J Cardiothorac Vasc Anesth 2014;28(3):652–60.
50. Baker WL, Radojevic J, Gluck JA. Systematic review of phosphodiesterase-5 inhibitor use in right ventricular failure following left ventricular assist device implantation. Artif Organs 2016;40(2):123–8.
51. Fitzpatrick JR 3rd, Frederick JR, Hiesinger W, et al. Early planned institution of biventricular mechanical circulatory support results in improved outcomes compared with delayed conversion of a left ventricular assist device to a biventricular assist device. J Thorac Cardiovasc Surg 2009;137(4):971–7.

52. Morgan JA, John R, Lee BJ, et al. Is severe right ventricular failure in left ventricular assist device recipients a risk factor for unsuccessful bridging to transplant and post-transplant mortality. Ann Thorac Surg 2004;77(3):859–63.
53. Leidenfrost J, Prasad S, Itoh A, et al. Right ventricular assist device with membrane oxygenator support for right ventricular failure following implantable left ventricular assist device placement. Eur J Cardiothorac Surg 2016;49(1):73–7.
54. Anderson MB, Goldstein J, Milano C, et al. Benefits of a novel percutaneous ventricular assist device for right heart failure: the prospective RECOVER RIGHT study of the Impella RP device. J Heart Lung Transpl 2015;34(12):1549–60.
55. Schmack B, Weymann A, Popov AF, et al. Concurrent left ventricular assist device (LVAD) implantation and percutaneous temporary RVAD support via CardiacAssist Protek-Duo TandemHeart to preempt right heart failure. Med Sci Monit Basic Res 2016;22:53–7.
56. Welp H, Sindermann JR, Deschka H, et al. Pulmonary bleeding during right ventricular support after left ventricular assist device implantation. J Cardiothorac Vasc Anesth 2016;30(3):627–31.
57. Krabatsch T, Stepanenko A, Schweiger M, et al. Alternative technique for implantation of biventricular support with HeartWare implantable continuous flow pump. ASAIO J 2011;57(4):333–5.
58. Strueber M, Meyer AL, Malehsa D, et al. Successful use of the HeartWare HVAD rotary blood pump for biventricular support. J Thorac Cardiovasc Surg 2010; 140(4):936–7.
59. Takeda K, Takayama H, Colombo PC, et al. Late right heart failure during support with continuous-flow left ventricular assist devices adversely affects post-transplant outcome. J Heart Lung Transpl 2015;34(5):667–74.

Device Management and Flow Optimization on Left Ventricular Assist Device Support

Inna Tchoukina, MD*, Melissa C. Smallfield, MD,
Keyur B. Shah, MD

KEYWORDS

- Left ventricular assist device • Heart failure • Mechanical circulatory support
- Pump thrombosis • Device parameters • Ramp study

KEY POINTS

- It is critical to know the device parameters while managing a patient on left ventricular assist device (LVAD) support.
- The LVAD flow depends on interaction between the pump and the native heart and is determined by speed of the pump rotation, preload at the pump inlet, and afterload at the pump outlet.
- The LVAD flow is directly proportional to the device speed (increases at higher speed settings) and inversely proportional to the pressure differential, ΔP, between the inflow and outflow (decreases as ΔP increases).
- Abnormal LVAD flow and pulsatility patterns help recognize LVAD-specific complications.
- Systematic analysis of LVAD parameters and echocardiographic and hemodynamic assessment allow for personalized optimization of LVAD flow.

INTRODUCTION

Left ventricular assist devices (LVAD) improve longevity, functional capacity, and quality of life in patients with refractory, end-stage (stage D) systolic heart failure.[1-3] The original concept of pulsatile flow pumps has been replaced with continuous-flow designs that allowed for miniaturization of the pump sizes, less device-associated infections, and improved device durability.[4] With less mechanical pump failures, long-term LVAD therapy has become a well-accepted reality to support patients until the time of heart transplantation, or as destination therapy for those ineligible for transplantation. As of December 2016, 17,634 patients received US Food and Drug

Disclosures: None.

Division of Cardiology, Department of Internal Medicine, Advanced Heart Failure and Transplantation, The Pauley Heart Center, Virginia Commonwealth University, 1200 East Broad Street, P.O. Box 980204, Richmond, VA 23298-0204, USA

* Corresponding author. Heart Failure and Transplantation, The Pauley Heart Center, Virginia Commonwealth University, MCV Campus, PO Box 980204, Richmond, VA 23298-0204.

E-mail address: inna.tchoukina@vcuhealth.org

Crit Care Clin 34 (2018) 453–463
https://doi.org/10.1016/j.ccc.2018.03.002
0749-0704/18/© 2018 Elsevier Inc. All rights reserved.

criticalcare.theclinics.com

Administration–approved continuous-flow LVADs in the Unites States alone with many more implants performed worldwide.[5,6] Currently, 3 continuous-flow LVADs are commercially available for clinical use in the United States: (a) HeartMate-II (Abbott Laboratories, Abbott Park, IL, USA), (b) HVAD (HeartWare Inc, Framingham, MA, USA), and (c) HeartMate-III (Abbott Laboratories, Abbott Park, IL, USA). Most acute care facilities are likely to encounter patients supported with LVADs, and it is imperative that providers of critical care are familiar with the hemodynamic principles of LVAD operation to ensure appropriate care.

In this article, the authors discuss the following:

- Principles of flow optimization in LVAD patients;
- Understanding of normal LVAD physiology and device interaction with the heart;
- Interpretation of LVAD parameters and their application to clinical assessment and patient care.

PRINCIPLES OF LEFT VENTRICULAR ASSIST DEVICE FUNCTION AND NORMAL LEFT VENTRICULAR ASSIST DEVICE PHYSIOLOGY

Contemporary LVADs consist of 3 basic components: an inflow cannula that attaches to the left ventricular (LV) apex or in its proximity and draws blood from the LV chamber into the device, the impeller that moves the volume of blood forward in parallel with native cardiac output, and an outflow tract that returns blood back into the vascular system via the proximal aorta.

The LVAD flow depends on a complex interaction between the pump and the native heart and is determined by the following 3 major components:

1. Programmed speed of the pump rotation,
2. Preload, or pressure/volume of blood available at the pump inlet, and
3. Afterload, or pressure at the pump outlet.

The speed of the device is directly proportional to the pump flow, that is, given a constant preload and afterload, the flow will increase at higher and decrease at lower LVAD speeds. The pressure difference between the pump inlet and outlet, in the absence of obstruction within the inflow cannula or the outflow tract, is termed "head pressure" or "ΔP." The flow of blood through the LVAD is inversely proportional

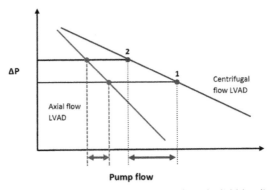

Fig. 1. Schematic representation of HQ curves of axial flow (*solid blue line*) and centrifugal flow (*solid red line*) LVADs, and impact of changing differential pressure ("ΔP") on the pump flow. As "ΔP" increases, the pump flow decreases (move from point 1 to point 2). The same change in "ΔP" will produce greater flow change in the centrifugal pump compared with the axial pump (*solid double-headed arrows*).

to the ΔP, that is, higher flows are generated as pressure differential declines (**Fig. 1**). Thus, the LVAD flow will either increase or decrease when the balance between the systemic blood pressure (afterload) and the LV pressure (preload) changes. That explains why the flow provided by the continuous-flow device is not entirely constant during the cardiac cycle. Preload increases during systole (augmented by native heart contraction), whereas systemic pressure remains relatively constant, which results in a drop of ΔP and an increase in pump flow. On the contrary, during diastole, the pump differential pressure increases and pump flow decreases.

Two conceptually different types of impellers exist to date: axial flow and centrifugal flow designs. In the axial flow pump, the impeller is a cylindrical shaft with 3 spiral blades; the impeller rotates along its axis inside the housing and "pushes" blood forward ("Archimedes screw"). The flow direction of the blood exiting the pump is coaxial to the flow direction entering the pump. The centrifugal flow impeller is shaped like a thick disk with blades that spins around its center of rotation and "propels" the blood outward; the blood enters the centrifuge through the inlet aligned with the rotational axis and leaves the housing perpendicular to the impeller (taking a 90° turn within the housing). Because of differences in design and engineering, the properties of the 2 types of impellers vary from one another. The mechanics and hydrodynamic performance (HQ) of axial versus centrifugal flow pumps are reviewed by Moazami and colleagues.[7] Briefly, the pressure-flow relationship of the LVAD at a given speed is described by the HQ curve, which is unique for each pump. In their recommended operating speed ranges, the axial flow LVADs tend to have steeper HQ curves, whereas the HQ curve of the centrifugal flow LVAD is flatter. The flat curve of centrifugal flow LVAD results in a wide change in flow for a small change in ΔP, whereas the steeper curve of an axial flow LVAD has a smaller variation of flow for the same change in ΔP (see **Fig. 1**). Consequently, an LVAD operating on a flatter segment of the HQ curve is more sensitive to afterload or high blood pressure (elevated systemic vascular resistance [SVR]) and will experience more significant drops in flow in a setting of poorly controlled hypertension. On the other hand, the flatter HQ curve may make the device less prone to over-decompressing the LV and causing suction in response to reduced LV preload (increased ΔP will generate less flow).

POWER, FLOW, AND PULSATILITY

When evaluating a patient, the LVAD parameters should be carefully reviewed in terms of absolute values as well as the trends for the individual patient. The device parameters that

Table 1
Device parameters in commercially available left ventricular assist devices

Device	Flow (L/min)[a]	Speed (rpm)[b]	Power (Watts)	Pulsatility
Heartmate-II	4–8	8800–10,000 (minimum 8600, maximum 12,000)	4–7	4–6
HVAD	4–7	2400–3200	3–7	Waveform pulsatility of 8–2 from peak to trough
Heartmate-III	3–6	5200–5800 (minimum 4800, maximum 6200)	3–7	1–4

[a] Maximal flow on LVAD is up to 10 L/min.
[b] Recommended clinical speed range on the device.

are clinically important are (a) pump speed, (b) power, (c) flow, and (d) pulsatility. The ranges of these parameters in the commercially available LVADs are shown in **Table 1**.

The speed in revolutions per minute is determined and programmed by a health care provider. The power consumption (watts) is a direct measure of the current and voltage applied to the motor. The flow (liters per minute) is calculated from the pump speed and power consumption. It is important to recognize that most of the currently available continuous-flow LVADs do not have flow sensors because of long-term reliability issues. Because the flow is calculated from the power consumption, these 2 parameters move in concert (as power increases, the flow will also increase, and vice versa). Although LVAD flow correlates with the measured cardiac output, the correlation coefficient is low, and the discrepancy between the LVAD flow and measured cardiac output is often seen, because the LVAD flow does not account for the output of the patient's left ventricle into the aorta.[8]

The variability in flow across a cardiac cycle is manifested by the pump pulsatility. It reflects how much cardiac output is provided by the patient's heart versus the pump. The pulsatility is expressed differently for HeartMate-II (axial flow), HeartMate-III, and HVAD (centrifugal flow) devices. For the HeartMate-II and HeartMate-III LVADs, the pulsatility index (PI) is used to quantify flow variation. It is a unitless measure calculated as beat-to-beat amplitude between the maximal flows and minimal flows averaged over 10 to 15 seconds and divided by the average flow according to the formula: (maximum flow – minimum flow)/average flow × 10. A larger difference in the peak instantaneous systolic and diastolic flows will be seen with higher LV contribution to the pump flow or less LVAD support relative to the residual LV contractility and will result in elevated PI. On the other hand, lower LV contractility or higher LVAD speed (more LVAD support) will reduce the numerator in the formula, and PI will be lower. Abrupt change in the PI is referred to as a PI event. Given a stable preload and afterload, changes in speed are inversely related to changes in PI: as the speed is increased, there is less native heart contribution and higher average flow, so the PI decreases. On HVAD, the pulsatility is displayed as a real-time flow waveform (**Fig. 2**A), which allows the operator to see systolic-diastolic variation of flow expressed numerically in liters per minute on the y-axis versus time on the x-axis. The implication of wider versus lower swing in the systolic-diastolic flows is similar to the high versus low PI as discussed above. Review of the flow waveform morphology offers an additional advantage of noting rhythm irregularities (as would be seen in atrial fibrillation) and other characteristic patterns (such as suction events, changes of flow with transitioning from supine to upright position, cough) (**Fig. 2**C).

A suction event is transient obstruction of the inflow cannula by ventricular myocardium typically caused by low preload. The suction alarms in LVADs are triggered by abrupt reductions of flow. In response, the device follows an algorithm to transiently reduce the speed to resolve the event.

Recognition of abnormal patterns on LVAD interrogation is an essential part of patient evaluation at bedside. Systematic analysis of pump parameters in a context of clinical presentation is necessary to diagnose complications and optimize LVAD function (**Fig. 3**).

DECREASED LEFT VENTRICULAR ASSIST DEVICE FLOW

Reduced LVAD flows and powers may be seen with low-speed operation or conditions that decrease LV preload or increase afterload (see **Fig. 3**A). Low LVAD preload states result in over-decompression of the LV and arise from several conditions. Hypovolemia from aggressive diuresis or acute bleeding is a common cause of reduced preload.

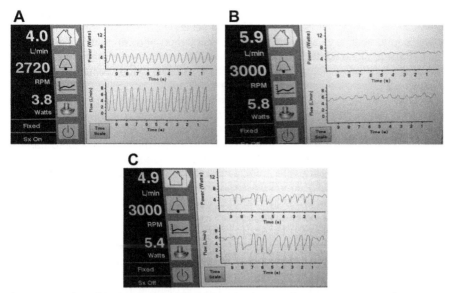

Fig. 2. Examples of high (*A*) and of low (*B*) pulsatility on the system monitor of an HVAD. The high pulsatility was observed in a patient with elevated Doppler-measured blood pressures. The low pulsatility pattern observed in (*B*) is associated with high or normal flows, which may be seen with high-speed operation, vasodilation, or severe AI. When moved from the supine to standing position (reduction in preload), this patient developed suction (*C*). The suction event resolved with reduction of the HVAD speed.

Compromised right ventricular (RV) function and elevated pulmonary vascular resistance also reduce blood return to the LVAD, thus reducing the LV filling pressure and causing a drop in pump flow. The pattern of low flow and low power combined with low PI with frequent PI events (on HeartMate-II and HeartMate-III LVADs), or low-amplitude pulsatility waveform and suction waveforms (on HVAD) may be indistinguishable from hypovolemic states but should raise suspicion for RV failure and trigger clinical investigation. Patients with a failing RV who undergo invasive hemodynamic evaluation will demonstrate elevated central venous pressure (CVP) in a setting of low pulmonary capillary wedge pressure (PCWP), and reduced measured cardiac

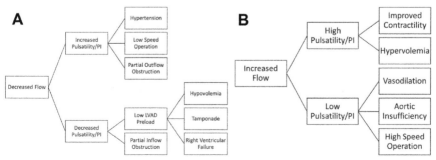

Fig. 3. Flow diagram highlighting typical causes of decreased (*A*) and increased (*B*) LVAD flow.

output. Imaging with bedside echocardiogram may confirm excessive decompression of the LV chamber (small "sucked in" LV) and severely dilated RV, leftward intraventricular septal shift, and severe tricuspid regurgitation (**Fig. 4**). The inflow cannula may come into close contact with the LV myocardium and trigger ventricular arrhythmias, which can further compromise RV function.[9] Atrial arrhythmias may contribute to RV dysfunction and should be corrected expeditiously, especially in the setting of symptomatic RV failure.[10] Inotropic therapies may be required to support RV contractility.[11] In addition, pulmonary vasodilation with inhaled nitric oxide or sildenafil may provide additional benefit by optimizing RV afterload and, therefore, improving RV output.[12,13] In severe cases, implantation of temporary right ventricular assist device may be necessary to ensure adequate systemic perfusion.

Findings of RV failure early after LVAD implantation should also raise the suspicion of pericardial tamponade. Echocardiography may be helpful, but acoustic windows early after surgery are often limited, and computed tomography (CT) of the chest may assist in making the correct diagnosis.[14]

A pattern of low LVAD flow associated with high pulsatility may identify distinct conditions. Hypertension increases afterload and therefore increases ΔP. Initially, hypertension leads to a more pronounced increase in ΔP during diastole. With reduced flow in diastole, the LVAD will display increased pulsatility or PI (see **Fig. 2**A). Severe hypertension can obliterate flow in both systole and diastole. Moreover, mean arterial pressure (MAP) in excess of 90 mm Hg has been shown to increase the risk of pump thrombosis and cerebrovascular events.[15–17] Careful titration of vasoconstrictive infusions to avoid high MAP and initiation of vasodilating medications when appropriate will help optimize pump flow and reduce the risk of complications.

Finally, low LVAD flow with high pulsatility may be simply a product of inappropriately low pump speed setting. Consider increasing the LVAD speed if invasive hemodynamic data suggest left heart failure (high wedge pressure, low cardiac output), and echocardiography demonstrates under-decompression the LV (increased LV chamber size, mitral regurgitation, frequent aortic valve opening).

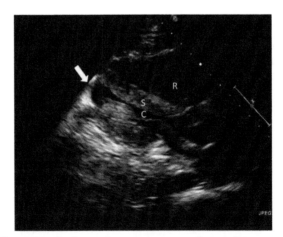

Fig. 4. Echocardiographic findings of a severe case of over-decompression of the left ventricle cavity (C). The inflow cannula (*white arrow*) is visualized in the parasternal long-axis view; the right ventricle (R) is dilated, and the interventricular septum (S) is bowed toward the left ventricle. This constellation of echocardiographic findings may occur in the setting of RV failure, hypovolemia, or high-speed operation.

Obstruction of the inflow cannula may occur as a result of thrombosis, tissue ingrowth, or cannula misalignment. Regardless of the cause, restriction of flow into the inflow cannula will result in diminished preload to the pump and reduced pump flow and power. Depending on whether the nature and degree of obstruction and LV contractility allow for augmentation of flow in systole, the pulsatility may be high, low, or unchanged. On the other hand, obstruction in the outflow tract may be caused by a kink in the graft, thrombosis, or, less commonly, external compression, and increases the afterload for the pump. As discussed above, high afterload will manifest itself as a low-flow and low-power situation on LVAD interrogation, again with variable degree of pulsatility. If suspected, imaging studies may shed light on the cause of abnormal pump findings and hemodynamics. Transthoracic echocardiography may not adequately visualize the inflow cannula because of imaging artifact, and Doppler interrogation of the flow into the cannula may be challenging due to difficulties aligning the ultrasonic beam with the axis of the blood flow. Likewise, distal segment of the outflow conduit and its anastomosis into the ascending aorta may be imaged using transthoracic technique, but more proximal segments of the outflow graft may not be well visualized with this imaging modality.[18] Thus, transesophageal or intravascular ultrasound may be needed to thoroughly evaluate both the inflow cannula and the outflow graft.[19] In addition, CT angiogram with 3-dimensional reconstruction allows for assessment of the course of the outflow conduit (**Fig. 5**).

INCREASED LEFT VENTRICULAR ASSIST DEVICE FLOW

High LVAD flow and power may be related to either increased preload, reduced afterload, or high-speed LVAD operation (see **Fig. 3**B).

The state of hypervolemia (elevated preload) reduces the ΔP leading to higher pump flow at the same pump speed. Clinically, the patient may have pulmonary congestion and peripheral edema despite higher than normal blood flow. Swan-Ganz catheter readings will show elevated CVP and PCWP and normal cardiac output. Echocardiographic evaluation may demonstrate failure to decompress the LV (increased LV

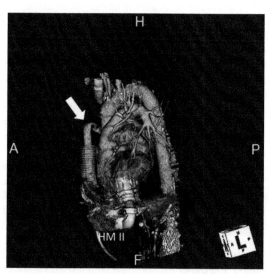

Fig. 5. CT scan with 3-dimensional reconstruction of the LVAD (HM-II) demonstrating obstruction due to a kink (*white arrow*) in the outflow graft. A, anterior (front); F, feet (bottom); H, head (top); P, posterior (back).

chamber size, mitral regurgitation, frequent aortic valve opening) and dilated inferior vena cava. Optimization of volume status with diuretics and/or ultrafiltration will help alleviate the congestion.

A unique condition of high flow and power occurs in the setting of severe aortic insufficiency (AI). As reported by Jorde and colleagues,[20] at least moderate AI develops in 37.6% of patients at 3 years after LVAD implantation. The blood delivered into the aorta by the LVAD recirculates back into the LV instead of reaching systemic circulation. Unlike AI of unsupported heart, which occurs in the diastolic phase of the cardiac cycle only, LVAD-associated AI may be continuous throughout both systole and diastole. As a result, LVAD preload is continuously increased throughout the cardiac cycle, and aortic pressure (afterload) drops rapidly in early diastole, resulting in persistently reduced ΔP, high pump flow, and low pulsatility (similar to waveform shown in **Fig. 2B**). Clinically, the patient with severe AI may present with symptoms of decompensated LV failure despite high LVAD flows. The AI is readily imaged on echocardiography, and right heart catheterization may confirm low measured cardiac output compared with LVAD displayed flow. Managing the LVAD speed with AI can be challenging. Lowering the LVAD speed may reduce the transvalvular gradient and amount of AI or result in increased LV filling pressure provoking exacerbation of heart failure.[21] Conversely, increasing the LVAD speed to "override" the AI may provide temporary relief in some patients. Surgical correction or transcatheter aortic valve implantation or closure is required for definitive treatment.

Vasodilation and low SVR can also lead to a high-flow low-pulsatility state. Causes of reduced SVR may include sepsis, overcorrected hypertension, and, less commonly, profound liver dysfunction, anaphylaxis, or adrenal insufficiency.

Pump thrombosis is a life-threatening complication of LVAD therapy and should be promptly recognized and treated. The hallmark of LVAD thrombosis is increased power with "power spikes" due to increased power consumption required to overcome the drag on the rotor. Because LVAD flow is calculated from the power consumption, the flows on the device interrogation are also "increased," whereas the actual LVAD output is reduced in the presence of large thrombus burden. The presentation may range from asymptomatic biochemical abnormalities (elevated lactate dehydrogenase [LDH] and free plasma hemoglobin concentration), to symptoms of hemolysis (darkening of urine), thromboembolism, stroke, acute decompensated heart failure, or cardiogenic shock. It has been shown that acute increase of LDH concentration is observed as early as 6 weeks before clinically apparent pump thrombosis, making it a sensitive marker for early detection of this devastating complication.[22] In the presence of significant pump malfunction, the echocardiogram will demonstrate inadequate LV decompression, inability to decrease LV diastolic dimension, and failure to "close" the aortic valve during the ramp study (discussed later).[23] Doppler interrogation of the inflow cannula and outflow graft may demonstrate abnormally low flow velocities or absence of blood flow. Intensification of anticoagulation regimen may occasionally resolve signs of hemolysis and normalize pump parameters. There are isolated case reports suggesting benefits of intravascular thrombolytic therapy in carefully selected patients. However, mortality associated with LVAD thrombosis is high and pump replacement is recommended if abnormalities persist despite aggressive anticoagulation. Emergent heart transplantation may also be considered in select cases.[15,22]

Finally, high pump flow with low pulsatility may be seen when the LVAD speed is set too high. In this scenario, the LVAD will compete with the left ventricle for available preload, shifting LVAD contractility down and leftward on the Frank-Starling curve. On echocardiography, the LV may look small (over-decompressed), and the aortic valve may fail to open. Suction events may occur and may be triggered by provocative maneuvers (orthostatic position change, cough, Valsalva maneuver) (see **Fig. 2**C).

An uncommon finding on LVAD interrogation is high pump flow in a setting of high pulsatility, suggesting some degree of myocardial recovery, which has been reported to occur in less than 1% of patients at 1 year.[24]

RAMP STUDY FOR ASSESSMENT OF DEVICE FUNCTION AND SPEED OPTIMIZATION

Assessment of interaction between LVAD and heart function at changing pump speeds is colloquially described as "ramp studies." These assessments may help diagnose device dysfunction or help identify optimal LVAD speed settings. These assessments can be done with echocardiography (echocardiography ramp study) or hemodynamic measurements (invasive ramp study) alone or in combination.

With increasing impeller speed, normal pump behavior is characterized by progressive decreases in LV dimensions, reduction in severity of mitral regurgitation, reduction in aortic valve leaflet excursion, or opening, and movement of the interventricular septum toward the posterior LV wall. Failure to demonstrate expected echocardiographic changes during the ramp study may identify flow obstruction within the pump (pump thrombosis), especially when combined with elevated LDH concentration (sensitivity of 100% and specificity of 93% with LDH level >5 times the upper limit of normal).[23]

Echocardiogram-guided ramp study is a readily available bedside tool to facilitate optimization of LVAD speed to attain most appropriate LV decompression (evidenced by improved LV diameter and minimized mitral regurgitation) while ensuring favorable RV geometry for more efficient RV function (neutral position of the interventricular septum avoiding leftward septal deviation, which results in increased RV strain and exacerbates tricuspid regurgitation).[25,26] In addition, some operators advocate for LVAD speed to allow intermittent aortic valve opening in order to prevent development of severe aortic regurgitation related to long-term continuous-flow LVAD support.[20]

Uriel and colleagues[27] recently demonstrated the value of invasive hemodynamic ramp study for LVAD speed optimization. It was shown that only 43% of stable LVAD patients managed using clinical and echocardiographic markers had normal right and left cardiac filling pressures, and only 23% had concomitant cardiac index greater than 2.0 L/min/m². Thus, right heart catheterization with LVAD speed titration is helpful to assess intravascular volume (guide diuretic therapy), LV decompression (adjustment of LVAD speed), SVR (optimization of afterload), pulmonary vascular resistance (need for pulmonary vasodilation), and RV function (indication for inotrope support in severe cases). In addition, hemodynamic ramp studies may identify abnormal pump behavior. Obstructed LVAD flow is suspected when PCWP fails to decrease and measured cardiac output fails to increase at higher LVAD speed and LVAD-derived flows. Likewise, in the presence of significant AI, ramp study will show minimal LV decompression and cardiac output response at higher LVAD speed.

EVIDENCE-BASED HEART FAILURE THERAPY

Reintroduction of guideline-directed heart failure medical therapy is recommended after LVAD implantation to facilitate myocardial recovery.[11] Furthermore, escalation of medications with vasodilatory properties may augment LVAD flow by reducing ΔP. In some patients, rapid changes in preload and/or afterload may unfavorably affect LVAD function and cause low-flow or suction events.

SUMMARY

Understanding normal physiology of LVADs and recognition of abnormal patterns of flow and pulsatility on device interrogation are essential for successful device and patient management. Despite differences in hemodynamic performance between the axial and centrifugal flow pumps, the basic principles of preload, afterload, and speed management are the same for all contemporary continuous-flow devices. Systematic analysis of LVAD parameters and echocardiographic and hemodynamic guidance allow for optimization and personalization of LVAD flow and detection of LVAD-related complications.

REFERENCES

1. Rose EA, Gelijns AC, Moskowitz AJ, et al. Long-term mechanical left ventricular assistance for end-stage heart failure. N Engl J Med 2001;345:1435–43.
2. Park SJ, Milano CA, Tatooles AJ, et al, HeartMate II Clinical Investigators. Outcomes in advanced heart failure patients with left ventricular assist devices for destination therapy. Circ Heart Fail 2012;5:241–8.
3. Aaronson KD, Slaughter MS, Miller LW, et al, HeartWare Ventricular Assist Device (HVAD) Bridge to Transplant ADVANCE Trial Investigators. Use of an intrapericardial, continuous-flow, centrifugal pump in patients awaiting heart transplantation. Circulation 2012;125:3191–200.
4. Slaughter MS, Rogers JG, Milano CA, et al, the HeartMate II Investigators. Advanced heart failure treated with continuous-flow left ventricular assist device. N Engl J Med 2009;361:2241–51.
5. Kirklin JK, Pagani FD, Kormos RL, et al. Eighth annual INTERMACS report: special focus on framing the impact of adverse events. J Heart Lung Transplant 2017;36:1080–6.
6. Kirklin JK, Cantor R, Mohacsi P, et al. First Annual IMACS Report: a global International Society for Heart and Lung Transplantation Registry for Mechanical Circulatory Support. J Heart Lung Transplant 2016;35:407–12.
7. Moazami N, Fukamachi K, Kobayashi M, et al. Axial and centrifugal continuous-flow rotary pumps: a translation from pump mechanics to clinical practice. J Heart Lung Transplant 2013;32:1–11.
8. Hasin T, Huebner M, Li Z, et al. Association of HeartMate II left ventricular assist device flow estimate with thermodilution cardiac output. ASAIO J 2014;60:513–8.
9. Garan AR, Levin AP, Topkara V, et al. Early post-operative ventricular arrhythmias in patients with continuous-flow left ventricular assist devices. J Heart Lung Transplant 2015;34:1611–6.
10. Oezpeker C, Zittermann A, Pühler T, et al. Permanent atrial fibrillation and 2 year clinical outcomes in patients with a left ventricular assist device implant. ASAIO J 2017;63:419–24.
11. Feldman D, Pamboukian SV, Teuteberg JJ, et al, International Society for Heart and Lung Transplantation. The 2013 International Society for Heart and Lung Transplantation Guidelines for mechanical circulatory support: executive summary. J Heart Lung Transplant 2013;32:157–87.
12. Argenziano M, Choudhri AF, Moazami N, et al. Randomized, double-blind trial of inhaled nitric oxide in LVAD recipients with pulmonary hypertension. Ann Thorac Surg 1998;65:340–5.
13. Tedford RJ, Hemnes AR, Russell SD, et al. PDE5A inhibitor treatment of persistent pulmonary hypertension after mechanical circulatory support. Circ Heart Fail 2008;1:213–9.

14. Carr CM, Jacob J, Park SJ, et al. CT of left ventricular assist devices. Radiogr Rev Publ Radiol Soc N Am Inc 2010;30:429–44.
15. Najjar SS, Slaughter MS, Pagani FD, et al, HVAD Bridge to Transplant ADVANCE Trial Investigators. An analysis of pump thrombus events in patients in the Heart-Ware ADVANCE bridge to transplant and continued access protocol trial. J Heart Lung Transplant 2014;33:23–34.
16. Teuteberg JJ, Slaughter MS, Rogers JG, et al, ADVANCE Trial Investigators. The HVAD left ventricular assist device: risk factors for neurological events and risk mitigation strategies. JACC Heart Fail 2015;3:818–28.
17. Rogers JG, Pagani FD, Tatooles AJ, et al. Intrapericardial left ventricular assist device for advanced heart failure. N Engl J Med 2017;376:451–60.
18. Stainback RF, Estep JD, Agler DA, et al, American Society of Echocardiography. Echocardiography in the management of patients with left ventricular assist devices: recommendations from the American Society of Echocardiography. J Am Soc Echocardiogr 2015;28:853–909.
19. Muller Moran HR, Kass M, Ravandi A, et al. Diagnosis of left ventricular assist device outflow graft obstruction using intravascular ultrasound. Circ Heart Fail 2016; 9(12) [pii:e003472].
20. Jorde UP, Uriel N, Nahumi N, et al. Prevalence, significance, and management of aortic insufficiency in continuous flow left ventricular assist device recipients. Circ Heart Fail 2014;7:310–9.
21. Holtz J, Teuteberg J. Management of aortic insufficiency in the continuous flow left ventricular assist device population. Curr Heart Fail Rep 2014;11:103–10.
22. Starling RC, Moazami N, Silvestry SC, et al. Unexpected abrupt increase in left ventricular assist device thrombosis. N Engl J Med 2014;370:33–40.
23. Uriel N, Morrison KA, Garan AR, et al. Development of a novel echocardiography ramp test for speed optimization and diagnosis of device thrombosis in continuous-flow left ventricular assist devices: the Columbia ramp study. J Am Coll Cardiol 2012;60:1764–75.
24. Topkara VK, Garan AR, Fine B, et al. Myocardial recovery in patients receiving contemporary left ventricular assist devices: results from the Interagency Registry for Mechanically Assisted Circulatory Support (INTERMACS). Circ Heart Fail 2016;9(7) [pii:e003157].
25. Holman WL, Bourge RC, Fan P, et al. Influence of left ventricular assist on valvular regurgitation. Circulation 1993;88:II309–18.
26. Topilsky Y, Hasin T, Oh JK, et al. Echocardiographic variables after left ventricular assist device implantation associated with adverse outcome. Circ Cardiovasc Imaging 2011;4:648–61.
27. Uriel N, Sayer G, Addetia K, et al. Hemodynamic ramp tests in patients with left ventricular assist devices. JACC Heart Fail 2016;4:208–17.

Complications of Durable Left Ventricular Assist Device Therapy

Sitaramesh Emani, MD

KEYWORDS

- Complications • Infection • Hemocompatibility • GI bleeding • Neurologic events

KEY POINTS

- Durable LVADs improve survival, functional capacity, and quality of life in advanced heart failure patients.
- The overall burden of complications from durable LVAD therapy has declined in the past 5 years.
- Complications related to the pump-patient interface include infections, acquired von Willebrand disease causing GI bleeding, pump thrombosis, and neurologic events.
- Patient-related complications include right ventricular failure, aortic valve insufficiency, and ventricular arrhythmias.
- It is hoped that improved patient selection and further design innovations will result in full biocompatibility of the LVAD, allowing patients to experience an excellent survival with a high quality of life that is free from complications.

INTRODUCTION

Durable left ventricular assist devices (LVADs) have consistently demonstrated utility in improving survival in patients with end-stage heart failure.[1] Ongoing use of LVADs, along with evolving technology, has resulted in ongoing improvements in survival with passing time.[2,3] In addition to survival benefit, LVADs have allowed for substantial improvements in quality of life for these patients.[4] Taken together, these benefits signal a likely increase in use of this therapy to treat heart failure, with some estimates suggesting that up to 250,000 patients within the United States alone could benefit from an LVAD.[5,6]

Despite improvements, complications from therapy still exist and can limit the potential benefits of an LVAD for any given patient. Registry data demonstrate the

Disclosure: Dr S. Emani is a paid consultant for the following companies: Abbott Laboratories, Medtronic, CHF Solutions, and Relypsa Pharmaceuticals.
Advanced Heart Failure and Cardiac Transplant, Division of Cardiovascular Medicine, The Ohio State University Wexner Medical Center, 473 West 12th Avenue, Suite 200 DHLRI, Columbus, OH 43221, USA
E-mail address: Sitaramesh.emani@osumc.edu

incidence of adverse events around 70% within 1 year of implant and a similarly high rate of rehospitalization within the first year.[3] Understanding these complications is critical to directing therapy, which may help mitigate long-term sequelae, and also help direct future investigations aimed to prevent the occurrence of complications.

VAD-related complications span a variety of forms, and can broadly be considered as aligning into three categories: (1) related to the pump and its accessories, such as pump or driveline or controller malfunction; (2) related to pump-patient interface, such as gastrointestinal bleeding (GIB) from acquired von Willebrand disease, neurologic events, infections, and pump thrombosis; and (3) related to the patient, such as arrhythmias, right heart failure, and aortic insufficiency. In the contemporary era, the total burden of complications on durable LVAD therapy is 29.2 events per 100 patient months. Although mechanical failure is possible and has been reported, manufacturing standards limit the incidence of these events, and are not reviewed in detail herein.

COMPLICATIONS RELATED TO PUMP-PATIENT INTERFACE
Infections

Infections are prevalent, occurring in nearly 30% of patients by 3 years of support, and can represent clinically significant complications.[3] They are the second most common cause of death in LVAD patients who survive the initial 6 months of support. They can range from superficial driveline infection (DLI) to pump pocket infection to frank sepsis or bloodstream infection (BSI). They often result in prolonged hospitalizations, multi-organ system failure, and sometimes death. They are not easy to eradicate and in addition to prolonged courses of multiple antibiotics, surgical debridement and rarely device replacement may be necessary.

With the evolution of LVAD design, observed rates of infection have significantly decreased. In the recent report on the newest generation of continuous centrifugal flow LVAD, Heartmate III (Abbott Industries, Pleasanton, CA), the DLI rate was 11.9%, and sepsis or BSI rate 9.3%.[3] Usually, BSI occurs in the perioperative period, whereas DLI are late onset infections. The average time to occurrence of DLI is 6 months after LVAD implantation. The risk factors for DLI are shown in **Box 1** and **Tables 1** and **2**. The most common organisms are bacterial skin organisms, such as *Staphylococcus epidermidis*, *Staphylococcus aureus*, and *Coryne bacterium*. DLI may remain superficial, but if not treated may spread along the driveline path into the pump pocket and abdominal wall, causing an abscess. Preoperative screening for colonization with multidrug-resistant bacteria can help identify high-risk patients for device-associated infection and facilitate preventative treatment.

Acquired von Willebrand Disease

Hemocompatibility is considered the spectrum of issues related to the interface between blood components with the VAD itself. Acquired von Willebrand disease is a unique, complex phenomenon that arises from hemocompatibility issues. As full-support devices, LVADs interface with nearly the entire blood volume of a patient on a continuous basis, creating a source of significant disruption to normal hematologic physiology, and biologic adaptation. As such, bleeding is the most frequent complication after LVAD implantation. Bleeding in the first 2 weeks after LVAD is usually related to the surgery. Risk factors for perioperative bleeding include hepatic dysfunction and postimplant right ventricular (RV) failure.

Early first-generation LVADs were pulsatile pumps that generated stroke volume with each cycle. The interface of synthetic materials with blood components was

---

Box 1
Complications after continuous-flow LVAD implantation

A. Related to pump and its accessories
   1. Driveline malfunction
   2. Controller malfunction
   3. Pump malfunction

B. Related to pump-patient interface
   1. Bleeding
      • Perioperative bleeding
      • Gastrointestinal bleeding from acquired von Willebrand disease
   2. Neurologic events
      • Ischemic stroke
      • Hemorrhagic stroke
   3. Infection
      • Driveline infection
      • Bloodstream infection
   4. Pump thrombosis

C. Related to the patient
   • Cardiac arrhythmia
   • Right heart failure
   • Valvular insufficiency

---

prothrombotic, similar to many other cardiac devices.[7] The properties of the materials used did not endothelialize, and as such, indefinite systemic anticoagulation was required in the form of an antiplatelet agent (ie, aspirin) and an oral vitamin K antagonist (VKA). Use of this combination while maintaining an appropriate level of anticoagulation (ie, achieving a goal international normalized ratio [INR] range) generally prevented the formation of thrombosis, although some thromboembolic consequences were noted.[8] Bleeding consequences were also infrequent, at a rate of 6.8 per 100 patient-years, which is similar to rates observed when systemic anticoagulation is instituted for other indications (eg, atrial fibrillation).[9,10] Although the rate of these complications was nonnegligible, they were considered acceptable. The limitation in this era of LVAD support was mechanical failure of the pump itself, making the approach less than ideal for long term support and necessitating the development of newer LVAD designs.[11]

LVAD designs evolved to continuous-flow devices, including axial flow devices, centrifugal pumps, and now fully magnetically levitated pumps. The first widespread use of continuous-flow devices came in the form of an axial flow pump (eg, HeartMate II, Abbott [Abbott Industries, Pleasanton, CA]), which uses a longitudinally

---

Table 1
Risk factors for driveline infection

Patient Factors	Surgical Technique	Wound Care Issues
• Age • Obesity • Poor nutrition • Diabetes • Chronic kidney disease • Preoperative colonization with bacteria	• Longer interfacial tunneling of the driveline • Anchoring and immobilization of driveline	• Trauma to the driveline • Noncompliance with wound care protocol • Lack of patient and/or caregiver education

Table 2
Adverse event rate in continuous-flow LVADs and BIVADs: April 2008–December 2016 (N = 17,632)

	1–3 mo		3–12 mo	
Complication	Number of Events	Rate (Events/100 Patient Months)	Number of Events	Rate (Events/100 Patient Months)
Infection	6552	13.63	4692	4.55
Bleeding	7810	16.24	4205	4.08
RV failure	238	0.57	276	1.17
Cardiac arrhythmia	5026	10.45	1359	1.92
Stroke	1162	2.42	1154	1.12
Thrombus	162	0.34	52	0.05

Abbreviations: BIVADs, biventricular assist devices; RV, right ventricular.

oriented impellar drawing blood through small gaps before returning it to systemic circulation.[12,13] Subsequently, centrifugal pumps (eg, HVAD, Medtronic [Medtronic, Inc, Minneapolis, MN]) were developed, which use a perpendicularly oriented rotary component reliant on blood components to serve as a hydrodynamic bearing.[14]

Continuous-flow pumps have resulted in increasing longevity of pumps, with some patients now on more than 10 years of support. However, increasing use of these pumps has seen an increase in bleeding complications, and in particular GIB, which is reported at 3 to 10 times higher in continuous-flow VAD patients. Investigation into the cause of GIB with continuous-flow VADs has uncovered a complex pathophysiology.[9]

Originally, the small blood gaps contained within these pumps were considered to be the trigger for GIB events. Hematologic homeostasis relies on the presence of von Willebrand factor (vWF). From a molecular standpoint, vWF is a reasonably large protein (205 kDa), and its active state depends on its three-dimensional confirmation.[15] Transit through continuous-flow VADs, with their small gaps, subjects vWF to shear forces that denature the protein structure and creates a functional deficiency of its active molecules.[16] A similar pattern was first described in aortic stenosis after an increased association with GIB was noted and eventually ascribed to vWF deficiency (Heyde syndrome).[15] Furthermore, standard operating ranges of continuous-flow pumps often lead to minimal opening of the aortic valve, creating a stenosis-like situation.

This pattern led to the theory that GIB in LVAD patients was related to vWF deficiency. Indeed, when vWF is measured in continuous-flow LVAD patients, levels are diminished.[16,17] However, follow-up studies failed to show a correlation between vWF levels and GIB. In fact, most continuous-flow LVAD patients have low levels of vWF, but a drop in levels does not discriminate between those patients who suffer a GIB and those who do not.[17]

Growing experience with GIB in the continuous-low LVAD population has uncovered arteriovenous malformations (AVMs) resulting from gastrointestinal angiodysplasia as an identifiable abnormality for patients who bleed.[18] AVMs are now suspected to be the primary source of GIB in many LVAD patients.[19] The high prevalence of AVM from angiodysplasia in this population compared with the normal population is intriguing, and may be the result of unique physiologic disturbances propagated by continuous flow. Evidence of these dysregulated processes is growing as a result of targeted investigations.

One pathway implicated in the formation of AVMs is the role of vascular endothelial growth factor. Vascular endothelial growth factor levels are increased by upregulation of signaling pathways, including transforming growth factor-β, which is elevated following implantation of continuous-flow LVADs.[20–23] Disruption of the transforming growth factor-β stimulation of vascular endothelial growth factor can occur through blockade of the angiotensin II pathway.[24–26] From this relationship, it follows that use of angiotensin receptor blockers may be protective against GIB, as was suggested by a retrospective analysis.[27] Other signaling pathways may be involved, such as hypoxia-inducible factors 1α and 2α, although the therapeutic implications of targeting these pathways is unclear.[28]

The median time to GIB is 33 days from surgery, although it can occur 18 months after LVAD implantation. The cumulative risk of GIB in continuous-flow LVADs at 1, 3, and 5 years is 21%, 27%, and 31%, respectively. GIB is the most common reason for 30-day readmission in LVAD patients. The site of GIB is often obscure and upper and lower endoscopies with small bowel follow through is frequently negative. Video capsule endoscopy may be helpful in identifying the location of GIB. In patients already suffering from the formation of AVMs and recurrent GIB, therapies aimed at preventing recurrent bleeds are not well described. Octreotide, a somatostatin analogue, is known to be effective in treating recurrent bleeding caused by vascular ectasia. In a case-controlled, retrospective analysis, use of octreotide correlated with a decreased incidence of recurrent GIB.[29] Improving understanding of tissue-level biologic changes resulting from the presence of VADs can help direct future studies aimed at treating and preventing these complications. As with many issues involving mechanically supported patients, prospective studies are lacking but are needed to improve outcomes.

Pump Thrombosis

Thrombosis in a continuous-flow LVAD is a serious, life-threatening complication. In addition, it may be a precursor for thromboembolic events. Historically, several clinical patient care decisions that were made have led to a rise in the incidence of this complication. Following the initial observation of increased GIB with continuous-flow LVADs, a variety of patient management changes made their way into clinical practice, not all of which was supported by data. Because of an early concern for vWF deficiency and a Heyde syndrome–style scenario, some practices advocated for the downtitration of pump speeds to allow intermittent opening of the aortic valve.[30] This strategy never proved to reduce GIB events, but may have inadvertently caused a prothrombotic environment within the LVAD itself. Because of the high RPMs of the impellars in the pumps, heat is generated by mechanical movement, especially in pump designs with fixed bearings. Constant flow of blood within the pump acts as a cooling mechanism to dissipate heat, which otherwise can trigger a thrombotic cascade. Extremely low speeds may diminish flow disproportionately compared with heat generation, leading to a net change of more unfavorable effects on blood components.[31,32] Furthermore, the desire to minimize anticoagulation as a contributing factor to bleeding led to changes in perioperative and chronic management strategies, including forgoing postoperative bridging with intravenous unfractionated heparin.[33]

From a chronic management standpoint, data emerged suggesting that the standardized management of VKAs with a target INR of 2 to 3 was not needed to prevent thrombosis, and instead INR ranges of 1.5 to 2 could be considered adequate.[34,35] Practices began to adjust target INR ranges, which may have been done inconsistently. Furthermore, studies examining time in therapeutic range for VKA therapy have demonstrated difficulty maintaining strict control, with only 20% of LVAD patients achieving at least 60% time in target range.[36] The unintended result of lower INR goals may have allowed patients to linger without adequate anticoagulation for prolonged periods of time, prompting a higher risk for thrombosis formation.

A subsequent analysis of adverse events reported an unexpected increase in thrombosis rates for continuous axial flow pumps, from an initial rate of 2.2% to 8.4% within 3 months of implant.[37] Concern over this increase prompted investigation into factors related to the increased risk of pump thrombosis. A striking finding from this analysis was an extremely variable rate of thrombosis among LVAD programs, suggesting implant techniques and management strategies could minimize the risk of thrombosis.[32] Further retrospective analysis identified the previously mentioned changes as specific contributors, which along with changes in surgical implant techniques that were adopted contemporaneously, were believed to contribute to changes in thrombosis rates.[38] There was no single major contributor among these factors.

To test the theory that combining optimal surgical and management strategies could decrease the risk of pump thrombosis, the Prevention of HeartMate II Pump Thrombosis Through Clinical Management study (PREVENT) was designed and conducted. In this study of 300 LVAD patients, attempted strict adherence to recommended best practices for continuous axial flow pump management was evaluated. This included good surgical technique for pump implantation, the use of bridging heparin postoperatively, avoidance of low pump speeds, and maintaining an INR goal of 2 to 2.5. The study demonstrated a reduction in pump thrombosis rate to 2.9% at 3 months and 4.8% and 6 months postimplant, both of which were similar to originally reported rates before 2011.[39]

Continuous axial flow pumps are not exclusively prone to pump thrombosis. Centrifugal pumps have thrombosis rates of 8.1% based on clinical trial data.[40] Because the adoption of centrifugal pumps occurred later than axial flow pumps, management strategies have not changed as much over time, and as a result, thrombosis rates have not been noted to change with increased use. Regardless, thrombosis and thromboembolic issues remain, including neurologic consequences. Factors that may affect thrombosis rates are likely similar to those affecting axial flow pumps, and similar best practice patterns are extended to the management of these pumps.

Newer generations of pumps have now been introduced with design feature that may help with issues of hemocompatibility. Fully magnetically levitated pumps are similar to centrifugal pumps on initial evaluation, but do not have physical bearings and have larger blood gaps within the pump housing. Conceptually, this allows for less shear on blood components and can prompt less prothrombotic changes. Additionally, the magnetic levitation design allows for rapid changes in impellar speed, which creates a "washing out" effect in blood gaps, preventing stasis.[41] Together, these features may account for the extremely low rate of pump thrombosis reported in initial clinical trials (none in the short-term cohort trial).[41] The low rate of thrombosis is promising, but the pump design has not eliminated all hemocompatibility adverse events; bleeding complications still occur in 30% of patients, half of which are GIB events.[41]

Although a reduction in thrombotic events was noted, it is unknown at this point if reduction in thrombosis risk through pump design will allow for future modification of baseline anticoagulation. Currently, magnetically levitated pumps still require standardized anticoagulation protocols with aspirin and VKAs, and the goal INR is considered to be 2 to 2.5. However, the mechanisms underlying bleeding, and in particular GIB, are complex and may not be mitigated by simply changing anticoagulation protocols.

Laboratory tests are helpful in the screening and diagnosis of pump thrombosis. LVAD thrombosis is often associated with hemolysis, which is detected by elevated levels of lactate dehydrogenase, indirect bilirubin, and plasma free hemoglobin levels. An echocardiographic ramp study is highly sensitive and specific for the diagnosis of LVAD thrombosis in axial flow pumps, but not centrifugal pumps. The role of computed tomography angiogram in the diagnosis of LVAD thrombosis is not clear.

There are no well-established guidelines for the treatment of LVAD thrombosis. Unfractionated heparin, thrombin inhibitors, local or systemic thrombolysis, and glycoprotein IIb/IIIa inhibitors alone or in combination have all been suggested. These therapies are associated with serious adverse effects, particularly bleeding. Often, an urgent transplantation or LVAD replacement is the only option (**Table 3**).

Neurologic Events

Neurologic events are additional adverse events that plague durable LVAD patients. The current rate of neurologic adverse events, including ischemic and hemorrhagic stroke, is approximately 10% at 1 year, and 25% at 4 years.[3] Neurologic events are most commonly thought to occur as a result of embolic phenomenon, including those that may emanate from the LVAD itself.[42] Risk factors for thromboembolic events include diabetes, full aortic cross-clamping with cardioplegic arrest during LVAD surgery, duration of LVAD support, and subtherapeutic INR (**Box 2**). The presence of atrial fibrillation is not associated with an increased risk of thromboembolic strokes. Given the presence of systemic anticoagulation, ischemic events can undergo hemorrhagic transformation. Additionally, centrifugal pumps are more sensitive to pump afterload, which clinically is measured as systemic hypertension.[43] Uncontrolled hypertension has been associated with an increased risk of thrombosis and thromboembolic events, and has prompted a need for better medical management of afterload.[40,44] Future investigations into risk factors for stroke may uncover additional risk factors. The hypothesis that cerebrovascular bed may undergo changes in the presence of continuous flow, similar to other vascular beds, may also predispose to neurologic events. Large vessels, such as the aorta, have already been shown to undergo histologic changes over time.[45] Perhaps, similar issues will be uncovered in smaller cerebral vessels, and may allow for targeted interventions.

Table 3
Pump thrombosis

Risk Factors	Diagnosis	Management

• Poor surgical implant technique
• Not using "bridging" heparin postoperatively
• Low pump speeds
• Subtherapeutic INR
	• LVAD diagnostics
	• Laboratory data
	  ○ LDH
	  ○ Plasma free hemoglobin
	  ○ Indirect bilirubin
	• Echocardiographic data
	  ○ Ramp study
	• CT angiogram
	• LVAD angiogram
		• Prevention
		  ○ Use of best practice guidelines
		• Treatment
		  ○ Increase antiplatelet therapy (dipyridamole, clopidogrel)
		  ○ Thrombin inhibitors (bivalirudin, argatroban)
		  ○ Local or systemic intravenous thrombolysis
		  ○ Intravenous glycoprotein IIb/IIIa inhibitors (abciximab, eptifibatide)
		  ○ Device exchange or explant
		  ○ Urgent cardiac transplantation

Abbreviations: CT, computed tomography; LDH, lactate dehydrogenase.

> **Box 2**
> **Risk factors for neurologic events**
>
> - Diabetes mellitus
> - Full aortic cross-clamping
> - Cardioplegic arrest during LVAD surgery
> - Duration of LVAD support
> - Subtherapeutic INR
> - Poor blood pressure control (in centrifugal devices)

COMPLICATIONS RELATED TO THE PATIENT
Heart Failure

Recurrent heart failure does represent one of post-LVAD complications, with potentially one in three patients likely to be rehospitalized for this reason after receiving a device.[46] Recurrent heart failure following LVAD placement, in the absence of pump problems (eg, thrombosis) illustrates the importance of intracardiac filling pressures in driving heart failure symptoms.[47] A functioning LVAD presumably augments cardiac output to an adequate degree; however, these patients can still experience dyspnea and volume retention. One series evaluating filling pressures in the presence of an LVAD showed that less than 60% of patients had optimized filling pressures following LVAD implantation.[48] For such patients, optimization of pump speed and concurrent evidence-based heart failure therapies can result in improved intracardiac pressures, resulting in an improved symptom burden.[49]

Although solid evidence does not exist to universally support the use of evidence-based heart failure therapies in LVAD patients, the conventional approach is to attempt the use of neurohormonal blockade when tolerated, as described in guidelines (with level of evidence C).[50] In practice systemic blood pressures may limit the aggressive use of heart failure therapies, although control of systemic hypertension is considered important for reducing the risk of neurologic events, particularly in patients on centrifugal devices. In scenarios where heart failure therapies can be added and titrated to maximal doses, improvements may be seen in native ventricular function, especially in certain populations.[51] Such improvements have led to ongoing explorations into the concept of myocardial recovery while on mechanical circulatory support. Ultimately, recovery of the myocardium to the point of LVAD explant may be the best way to mitigate the risk for heart failure on VAD therapy.[52]

Right Ventricular Failure

The prevention and treatment of RV failure during LVAD therapy is discussed separately in great detail in this issue. RV function is of critical importance in LVAD-supported patients, both immediately postoperatively and during chronic support. Acute RV failure is a major cause of morbidity and mortality during the index hospitalization and is underscored by the lack of reliable therapies to treat it effectively.[53] It is seen in about 11% of patients after LVAD implantation. Most notably, the absence of reliable medical therapy and approved durable RV support devices limit options to temporary devices, off-label use of durable VADs designed to support the left ventricle, or implantation of a total artificial heart. Unfortunately, none of these options have consistently demonstrated good outcomes.[3]

Late RV failure has proven equally difficult to treat, particularly because the cause is incompletely understood.[54] In many cases, the pathobiologic process that affected the LV likely affected the RV pre-LVAD, either at the tissue level or secondarily through hemodynamic insult. Current LVAD technology does not truly adjust itself to modulate cardiac output, and as a result, a constant, continuous flow is maintained independent of physiologic need and autoregulatory mechanisms. Whether or not this continuous flow rate contributes to late RV failure is unknown, but the RV may not have the ability to compensate for this unrelenting flow rate, which may result in remodeling and failure after prolonged periods of support.[53] Similar to acute RV failure therapeutic options are limited for late RV failure unless transplant is in consideration and available. Ultimately, late RV failure leads to death on chronic support.[3]

Valvular Insufficiency

Both mitral and aortic valve insufficiency can be seen after LVAD support. Mitral insufficiency, if severe preoperatively, may require surgical repair at the time of LVAD implantation. In general, functional mitral regurgitation present preoperatively improves immediately following LV unloading with an LVAD, with continued improvement as the LV progressively reverse remodels on durable support. Persistent residual, significant mitral regurgitation is often associated with RV dysfunction and pulmonary hypertension and confers a risk for rehospitalization on LVAD support and death. Optimization of LVAD parameters, aggressive diuresis, and afterload reduction should be considered in patients with persistent residual mitral regurgitation on LVAD support.

Aortic valve insufficiency can occur in 11% to 40% of patients supported with an LVAD. The mechanism is multifactorial and includes variation in pressure and flow in the aortic root, incorrect angle between the outflow graft and the aorta that results in weakening and dilatation of the aortic root and incomplete coaptation of the valve leaflets, and degeneration of the aortic root caused by high-velocity, high-diastolic pressures and shear stress. The presence of aortic insufficiency affects pump performance and can result in worsening heart failure. Fortunately, aortic insufficiency is rarely severe and does not require surgical intervention.

Cardiac Arrhythmias

Atrial arrhythmias are common perioperatively and are usually responsive to antiarrhythmic therapy or electrical cardioversion. Some patients with preoperative persistent atrial fibrillation may continue to remain in atrial fibrillation postoperatively. The presence of persistent atrial fibrillation is not associated with issues related to pump performance, or increased risk of pump thrombosis or thromboembolic events in patients on continuous-flow LVAD support.[3]

Despite a low incidence, mortality among LVAD patients with ventricular arrhythmias (VA) is twice as high as seen among those without VA. In particular, VA in the first week postoperatively is associated with a high mortality risk.[3] Monomorphic ventricular tachycardia is the most common VA observed after LVAD implantation. Most patients with VA present with palpitations, presyncope or syncope, worsening dyspnea, or heart failure. Death occurs when the LVAD output drops from decreased preload caused by RV failure. VA can occur in patients with and without ischemia and the cause is not always clear. Apical scarring from placement of the outflow cannula and ventricular suction events are potential risk factors. Treatment of VA is difficult, particularly when antiarrhythmic drugs and β-blockers are ineffective. There is general consensus that automatic implantable cardioverter defibrillator, if present preoperatively (which is often the case), should be continued. Select patients are candidates for either radiofrequency ablation or cryoablation and further studies are needed to analyze the sustained benefit of this therapy.

SUMMARY

The occurrence of LVAD-related complications continues to be a limitation of this life-saving therapy. It is hoped that improving the understanding of risk factors and mechanisms that underlie these events will pave the way to their reduction, whether that be through improved pump design, management strategies, or implementation of therapies that prevent their development. Although complications are common, thankfully not all of them result in worsening quality of life. In a recent study, LVAD patients who had suffered a significant adverse event, including bleeding or stroke, significantly improved their functional status and quality of life when compared with preimplant levels. Quality of life measures were not significantly different between patients who had an adverse event and those that were event-free.[55] Although this may indicate a lack of sensitivity in the metrics used, the findings more than likely indicate that in appropriate candidates with advanced heart failure, LVAD therapy uniformly improves quality of life and survival and should be considered despite ongoing risks from therapy.

REFERENCES

1. Rose EA, Gelijns AC, Moskowitz AJ, et al. Long-term use of a left ventricular assist device for end-stage heart failure. N Engl J Med 2001;345(20):1435–43.
2. Jorde UP, Kushwaha SS, Tatooles AJ, et al. Results of the destination therapy post-food and drug administration approval study with a continuous flow left ventricular assist device: a prospective study using the INTERMACS registry (interagency registry for mechanically assisted circulatory support). J Am Coll Cardiol 2014;63(17):1751–7.
3. Kirklin JK, Pagani FD, Kormos RL, et al. Eighth annual INTERMACS report: special focus on framing the impact of adverse events. J Heart Lung Transplant 2017;36(10):1080–6.
4. Rogers JG, Aaronson KD, Boyle AJ, et al. Continuous flow left ventricular assist device improves functional capacity and quality of life of advanced heart failure patients. J Am Coll Cardiol 2010;55(17):1826–34.
5. Miller LW, Guglin M. Patient selection for ventricular assist devices: a moving target. J Am Coll Cardiol 2013;61(12):1209–21.
6. Gordon RJ, Weinberg AD, Pagani FD, et al. Prospective, multicenter study of ventricular assist device infections. Circulation 2013;127(6):691–702.
7. Alba AC, Delgado DH. The future is here: ventricular assist devices for the failing heart. Expert Rev Cardiovasc Ther 2009;7(9):1067–77.
8. Kirklin JK, Naftel DC, Kormos RL, et al. Third INTERMACS annual report: the evolution of destination therapy in the United States. J Heart Lung Transplant 2011; 30(2):115–23.
9. Crow S, John R, Boyle A, et al. Gastrointestinal bleeding rates in recipients of nonpulsatile and pulsatile left ventricular assist devices. J Thorac Cardiovasc Surg 2009;137(1):208–15.
10. Shoeb M, Fang MC. Assessing bleeding risk in patients taking anticoagulants. J Thromb Thrombolysis 2013;35(3):312–9.
11. Cheng A, Williamitis CA, Slaughter MS. Comparison of continuous-flow and pulsatile-flow left ventricular assist devices: is there an advantage to pulsatility? Ann Cardiothorac Surg 2014;3(6):573–81.

12. Griffith BP, Kormos RL, Borovetz HS, et al. HeartMate II left ventricular assist system: from concept to first clinical use. Ann Thorac Surg 2001;71(3 Suppl): S116–20 [discussion: S114–6].

13. Miller LW, Pagani FD, Russell SD, et al. Use of a continuous-flow device in patients awaiting heart transplantation. N Engl J Med 2007;357(9):885–96.

14. Wieselthaler GM, O Driscoll G, Jansz P, et al, HVAD Clinical Investigators. Initial clinical experience with a novel left ventricular assist device with a magnetically levitated rotor in a multi-institutional trial. J Heart Lung Transplant 2010;29(11): 1218–25.

15. Loscalzo J. From clinical observation to mechanism: Heyde's syndrome. N Engl J Med 2012;367(20):1954–6.

16. Meyer AL, Malehsa D, Bara C, et al. Acquired von Willebrand syndrome in patients with an axial flow left ventricular assist device. Circ Heart Fail 2010;3(6): 675–81.

17. Meyer AL, Malehsa D, Budde U, et al. Acquired von Willebrand syndrome in patients with a centrifugal or axial continuous flow left ventricular assist device. JACC Heart Fail 2014;2(2):141–5.

18. Demirozu ZT, Radovancevic R, Hochman LF, et al. Arteriovenous malformation and gastrointestinal bleeding in patients with the HeartMate II left ventricular assist device. J Heart Lung Transplant 2011;30(8):849–53.

19. Wever-Pinzon O, Selzman CH, Drakos SG, et al. Pulsatility and the risk of nonsurgical bleeding in patients supported with the continuous-flow left ventricular assist device HeartMate II. Circ Heart Fail 2013;6(3):517–26.

20. Welp H, Rukosujew A, Tjan TD, et al. Effect of pulsatile and non-pulsatile left ventricular assist devices on the renin-angiotensin system in patients with end-stage heart failure. Thorac Cardiovasc Surg 2010;58(Suppl 2):S185–8.

21. Shao ES, Lin L, Yao Y, et al. Expression of vascular endothelial growth factor is coordinately regulated by the activin-like kinase receptors 1 and 5 in endothelial cells. Blood 2009;114(10):2197–206.

22. Ferrari G, Cook BD, Terushkin V, et al. Transforming growth factor-beta 1 (TGF-beta1) induces angiogenesis through vascular endothelial growth factor (VEGF)-mediated apoptosis. J Cell Physiol 2009;219(2):449–58.

23. Bertolino P, Deckers M, Lebrin F, et al. Transforming growth factor-beta signal transduction in angiogenesis and vascular disorders. Chest 2005;128(Suppl 6): 585S–90S.

24. Brooke BS, Habashi JP, Judge DP, et al. Angiotensin II blockade and aortic-root dilation in Marfan's syndrome. N Engl J Med 2008;358(26):2787–95.

25. Langham RG, Kelly DJ, Gow RM, et al. Transforming growth factor-beta in human diabetic nephropathy: effects of ACE inhibition. Diabetes Care 2006;29(12): 2670–5.

26. el-Agroudy AE, Hassan NA, Foda MA, et al. Effect of angiotensin II receptor blocker on plasma levels of TGF-beta 1 and interstitial fibrosis in hypertensive kidney transplant patients. Am J Nephrol 2003;23(5):300–6.

27. Houston BA, Schneider AL, Vaishnav J, et al. Angiotensin II antagonism is associated with reduced risk for gastrointestinal bleeding caused by arteriovenous malformations in patients with left ventricular assist devices. J Heart Lung Transplant 2017;36(4):380–5.

28. Yamakawa M, Liu LX, Date T, et al. Hypoxia-inducible factor-1 mediates activation of cultured vascular endothelial cells by inducing multiple angiogenic factors. Circ Res 2003;93(7):664–73.

29. Shah KB, Gunda S, Emani S, et al. Multicenter evaluation of octreotide as secondary prophylaxis in patients with left ventricular assist devices and gastrointestinal bleeding. Circ Heart Fail 2017;10(11):1–7.

30. Cowger J, Pagani FD, Haft JW, et al. The development of aortic insufficiency in left ventricular assist device-supported patients. Circ Heart Fail 2010;3(6):668–74.

31. Uriel N, Han J, Morrison KA, et al. Device thrombosis in HeartMate II continuous-flow left ventricular assist devices: a multifactorial phenomenon. J Heart Lung Transplant 2014;33(1):51–9.

32. Stulak JM, Maltais S. A different perspective on thrombosis and the HeartMate II. N Engl J Med 2014;370(15):1467–8.

33. Slaughter MS, Naka Y, John R, et al. Post-operative heparin may not be required for transitioning patients with a HeartMate II left ventricular assist system to long-term warfarin therapy. J Heart Lung Transplant 2010;29(6):616–24.

34. Menon AK, Gotzenich A, Sassmannshausen H, et al. Low stroke rate and few thrombo-embolic events after HeartMate II implantation under mild anticoagulation. Eur J Cardiothorac Surg 2012;42(2):319–23 [discussion: 323].

35. Boyle AJ, Russell SD, Teuteberg JJ, et al. Low thromboembolism and pump thrombosis with the HeartMate II left ventricular assist device: analysis of outpatient anti-coagulation. J Heart Lung Transplant 2009;28(9):881–7.

36. Boehme AK, Pamboukian SV, George JF, et al. Anticoagulation control in patients with ventricular assist devices. ASAIO J 2017;63(6):759–65.

37. Starling RC, Moazami N, Silvestry SC, et al. Unexpected abrupt increase in left ventricular assist device thrombosis. N Engl J Med 2014;370(1):33–40.

38. Taghavi S, Ward C, Jayarajan SN, et al. Surgical technique influences HeartMate II left ventricular assist device thrombosis. Ann Thorac Surg 2013;96(4):1259–65.

39. Maltais S, Kilic A, Nathan S, et al. PREVENtion of HeartMate II pump thrombosis through clinical management: the PREVENT multi-center study. J Heart Lung Transplant 2017;36(1):1–12.

40. Najjar SS, Slaughter MS, Pagani FD, et al. An analysis of pump thrombus events in patients in the HeartWare ADVANCE bridge to transplant and continued access protocol trial. J Heart Lung Transplant 2014;33(1):23–34.

41. Mehra MR, Naka Y, Uriel N, et al. A fully magnetically levitated circulatory pump for advanced heart failure. N Engl J Med 2017;376(5):440–50.

42. Morgan JA, Brewer RJ, Nemeh HW, et al. Stroke while on long-term left ventricular assist device support: incidence, outcome, and predictors. ASAIO J 2014;60(3):284–9.

43. Moazami N, Fukamachi K, Kobayashi M, et al. Axial and centrifugal continuous-flow rotary pumps: a translation from pump mechanics to clinical practice. J Heart Lung Transplant 2013;32(1):1–11.

44. Lampert BC, Eckert C, Weaver S, et al. Blood pressure control in continuous flow left ventricular assist devices: efficacy and impact on adverse events. Ann Thorac Surg 2014;97(1):139–46.

45. Ambardekar AV, Hunter KS, Babu AN, et al. Changes in aortic wall structure, composition, and stiffness with continuous-flow left ventricular assist devices: a pilot study. Circ Heart Fail 2015;8(5):944–52.

46. Hasin T, Marmor Y, Kremers W, et al. Readmissions after implantation of axial flow left ventricular assist device. J Am Coll Cardiol 2013;61(2):153–63.

47. Fonarow GC, Heywood JT, Heidenreich PA, et al, ADHERE Scientific Advisory Committee and Investigators. Temporal trends in clinical characteristics, treatments, and outcomes for heart failure hospitalizations, 2002 to 2004: findings

from Acute Decompensated Heart Failure National Registry (ADHERE). Am Heart J 2007;153(6):1021–8.

48. Uriel N, Sayer G, Addetia K, et al. Hemodynamic ramp tests in patients with left ventricular assist devices. JACC Heart Fail 2016;4(3):208–17.

49. Imamura T, Chung B, Nguyen A, et al. Clinical implications of hemodynamic assessment during left ventricular assist device therapy. J Cardiol 2018;71(4): 352–8.

50. Feldman D, Pamboukian SV, Teuteberg JJ, et al. The 2013 international society for heart and lung transplantation guidelines for mechanical circulatory support: executive summary. J Heart Lung Transplant 2013;32(2):157–87.

51. Simon MA, Primack BA, Teuteberg J, et al. Left ventricular remodeling and myocardial recovery on mechanical circulatory support. J Card Fail 2010;16(2): 99–105.

52. Drakos SG, Pagani FD, Lundberg MS, et al. Advancing the science of myocardial recovery with mechanical circulatory support: a working group of the National, Heart, Lung, and Blood Institute. JACC Basic Transl Sci 2017;2(3):335–40.

53. Lampert BC, Teuteberg JJ. Right ventricular failure after left ventricular assist devices. J Heart Lung Transplant 2015;34(9):1123–30.

54. Takeda K, Takayama H, Colombo PC, et al. Incidence and clinical significance of late right heart failure during continuous-flow left ventricular assist device support. J Heart Lung Transplant 2015;34(8):1024–32.

55. Cowger JA, Naka Y, Aaronson KD, et al. Quality of life and functional capacity outcomes in the MOMENTUM 3 trial at 6 months: a call for new metrics for left ventricular assist device patients. J Heart Lung Transplant 2018;37(1):15–24.

Challenges and Future Directions in Left Ventricular Assist Device Therapy

Manreet K. Kanwar, MD[a],*, Stephen Bailey, MD[b],
Srinivas Murali, MD[b]

KEYWORDS

- Left ventricular assist device • Future challenges • End-stage heart failure
- Mechanical circulatory support

KEY POINTS

- Left ventricular assist devices (LVADs) are being increasingly used in patients with end-stage heart failure, both as bridge to transplantation and as destination therapy.
- LVADs offer longer survival and improvements in quality of life in carefully selected patients, but not without risk of adverse events and social burdens.
- LVAD therapy is expensive and associated with significant resource utilization.
- Technologic evolution will lessen adverse events and perhaps facilitate adoption of this therapy in newer patient cohorts.
- Optimal cost-effective use of this expensive, risky therapy in heart failure will however require availability of reliable risk stratification tools.

INTRODUCTION

Left ventricular assist devices (LVADs) are being increasingly used in the management of patients with end-stage heart failure (HF).[1] Initially introduced as temporary mechanical circulatory support (MCS) devices for postcardiotomy failure, LVADs have now emerged as a lead option to bridge patients to transplantation (BTT), supporting patients for increasing lengths of time.[2] The evolution of LVADs over the last 5 decades has seen progression from pulsatile flow pumps to continuous flow devices, and within that category from axial flow to centrifugal flow (**Box 1**). Currently, there are 3 devices used commercially for the BTT indication, and 2 devices approved as destination therapy

Disclosure: None.
[a] Section of Heart Failure/Transplant/MCS and Pulmonary Hypertension, Cardiovascular Institute, Allegheny Health Network, Temple University School of Medicine, 320 East North Avenue, 16th Floor ST, Pittsburgh, PA 15212, USA; [b] Department of Cardiothoracic Surgery, Cardiovascular Institute, Allegheny Health Network, 320 East North Avenue, Pittsburgh, PA 15212, USA
* Corresponding author.
E-mail address: manreet.kanwar@ahn.org

Crit Care Clin 34 (2018) 479–492
https://doi.org/10.1016/j.ccc.2018.03.010
0749-0704/18/© 2018 Elsevier Inc. All rights reserved.

Box 1
Evolution of mechanical circulatory support in the United States

Decade	Evolution of MCS
1960	• National Institutes of Health (NIH) forms Artificial Heart Program • First implantable pneumatic LVAD by DeBakey
1970	• NIH proposal for long-term LVAD
1980	• First TAH use for permanent support (Jarvik-7) • First LVAD use as BTT
1990	• US Food and Drug Administration (FDA) approves PF-LVAD (HeartMate XVE) for BTT
2000	• FDA approves PF-LVAD (HeartMate XVE) for DT • INTERMACS Registry established • FDA approves CF-LVAD (HeartMate II) for BTT • FDA approves Syncardia TAH for BTT
2010	• FDA approves CF-LVAD (axial flow-HeartMate II) for DT • FDA approves CF-LVAD (centrifugal flow-HVAD) for BTT • ROADMAP trial shows functional improvement in INTERMACS profiles 4–7 with CF-LVAD • FDA approves CF-LVAD (centrifugal flow-HVAD) for DT • FDA approves CF-LVAD (centrifugal flow-HeartMate III) for BTT • Remission from Stage D HF (RESTAGE HF) trial to determine if LVAD support can result in sufficient improvement in ventricular function to facilitate device explantation

Abbreviation: TAH, total artificial heart.

(DT) devices for those patients with end-stage HF who are ineligible for heart transplantation (HT) (**Fig. 1**). Bridge to decision (BTD) therapy allows LVADs to support patients who are not currently qualified for HT but may become so in the future. Last, bridge to recovery (BTR) therapy intends to provide extended hemodynamic support to allow patients time for myocardial recovery and eventual LVAD explant.

The current generation pumps offer several significant improvements in pump design, size, and durability compared with first-generation devices. These innovations have allowed for longer, event-free support options for patients with improved quality of life. Current survival for patients implanted with a continuous flow LVAD (CF-LVAD) is 81% at 1 year, which is similar to the survival of a United Network for Organ Sharing (UNOS) status 2 patient on the HT waiting list, and 59% at 3 years (**Tables 1** and **2**).[1,3] Patients report increased exercise capacity and improved quality of life while being supported with durable LVADs. However, despite improvement in pump technology, several LVAD recipients continue to face risk of morbidity and mortality caused by bleeding, right HF, infections, pump thrombosis, neurologic events, and multiorgan failure.[4] These risks present several challenges and also opportunities for improvement with further advances in technology. Improvements in the near future are focused on improving clinical management strategies, introduction of pulsatility, use of more biocompatible materials, and development of full implantable systems.

FOCUS ON EVOLVING INDICATIONS

Over the years, the landscape of candidates being considered for durable LVAD support has evolved.[2] As the number of patients with end-stage HF in the United States continues to increase, HT continues to be limited to about 2000 per year because of donor availability constraints. Currently, there are more than 6 million people with HF in the United States, of whom an estimated 500,000 patients have advanced HF. Half of the HF population has preserved left ventricular ejection fraction (HFpEF) and are not

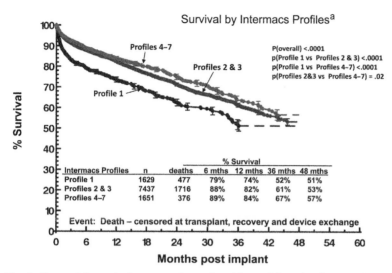

Fig. 1. Parametric survival curve and associated hazard function from INTERMACS Registry for CF-LVADs, including both isolated LVADs and biventricular assist device (BiVAD). The dashed lines indicate 70% confidence limits. [a] 9 patients with unspecified patient profile at time if implant. (*From* Kirklin JK, Pagani FD, Kormos RL, et al. Eighth annual INTERMACS report: special focus on framing the impact of adverse events. J Heart Lung Transplant 2017;36(10):1082; with permission.)

suitable for LVAD therapy based on current evidence. Unfortunately, morbidity and survival for HFpEF patients mirrors that observed in patients with reduced ejection fraction (HFrEF).[5] There is preliminary evidence that LVAD support is feasible in patients with restrictive cardiomyopathy and HFpEF, particularly those with larger end-diastolic and end-systolic dimensions.[6] Further studies are needed to define if LVAD support is an effective therapeutic option for the large universe of patients with end-stage HFpEF.

With a wider availability of LVADs, an increasing number of patients who are receiving implants are in Interagency Registry for Mechanically Assisted Circulatory Support (INTERMACS) profiles 2 and 3, with a good number in INTERMACS profile 4. In fact, from 2013 to 2016, more LVAD implants were performed in INTERMACS profile 4 to 7, compared with INTERMACS profile 1. Survival in INTERMACS profiles 2 to 3 and 4 to 7 remains superior to INTERMACS profile 1 (**Fig. 2**). Compared with optimal medical therapy, patients in INTERMACS profile 4 to 7 are more likely to have improvement in submaximal exercise capacity, health-related quality of life, and 2-year actuarial survival with LVAD support, despite a higher cumulative adverse event rate (**Fig. 3**).[7] The improvements were particularly striking in INTERMACS profile 4 patients. The key adverse events decreased in the LVAD group after 1 year, favoring risk-benefit of elective LVAD therapy in INTERMACS profiles 4 to 7. Based on these data, it is expected that increasing numbers of patients in INTERMACS profile 4 to 7 will receive LVAD therapy in the future. Furthermore, comorbidities are frequently present in patients with advanced stage D HFrEF, and their prevalence continues to increase. Because the presence of comorbidities may independently increase the risk of LVAD surgery, it is important that decisions regarding LVAD implantation are made when patients are in INTERMACS profile 4 to 7, rather than 1 to 3.

Table 1
Comparison of LVAD technology

Features	Heartmate XVE	Heartmate 2	HeartWare HVAD	Heartmate 3
Flow	Pulsatile (PF)	Continuous (CF) axial	Continuous (CF) centrifugal	Continuous (CF) centrifugal
Pump Design	Pusher plate	Internal rotor	Impellar	Internal rotor
Mechanical bearing	Yes	Yes	No (combined magnetic and hydrodynamic levitation)	No (fully magnetic levitation)
Inflow cannula from LV apex	Yes (with inflow valve)	Yes (with inlet stator)	Yes (short inflow cannula)	Yes (short inflow cannula)
Outflow graft to aorta	Yes (with outflow valve)	Yes (with outlet stator)	Yes	Yes
Pump placement	Abdomen (pre-peritoneal)	Abdomen (pre-peritoneal)	Thorax (intra-pericardial)	Thorax
Per-cutaneous Driveline	Yes	Yes	Yes	Yes
External system controller	Yes	Yes	Yes	Yes
Power source	External battery pack	External battery pack	External battery pack	External battery pack
Clinical use in 2018	FDA approved for BTT and DT (Not used)	FDA approved for BTT and DT	FDA approved for BTT and DT	FDA approved for short-term use

Abbreviations: CF, continuous flow; FDA, Food and Drug administration; PF, pulsatile flow.

Table 2
Comparison of major clinical trials evaluating LVADs in advanced heart failure

Parameters	REMATCH	Heartmate 2 BTT	Heartmate 2 DT	ADVANCE	ENDURANCE	MOMENTUM 3 Short-Term	MOMENTUM 3 Long-Term
Comparator groups	HM XVE vs OMT	HM 2 vs OMT	HM 2 vs HM XVE	HVAD vs.commercially available LVADs	HVAD vs HM 2	HM 3 vs HM 2	HM 3 vs HM 2
Design	Randomized (1:1)	Non-randomized	Randomized (2:1)	Non-randomized	Randomized (2:1)	Randomized (1:1)	Randomized (1:1)
No. of patients	129	133	200	140	446	294	366
Patient profile	TX ineligible, NYHA IV	TX listed, NYHA IV	TX ineligible, NYHA III & IV	TX listed, NYHA IV	TX ineligible, INTERMACS 1–4	TX listed and ineligible, INTERMACS 1–4	TX listed and ineligible, INTERMACS 1–4
Primary endpoint	Improved survival at 1 & 2 y	Improved survival at 6 mo	Improved event free survival at 2 y	Non-inferiority in survival at 1 y	Non-inferiority in event free survival at 2 y	Improved event free survival at 6 mo	Improved event free survival at 2 y
Functional Capacity	Improved	Improved	Improved in both groups	Improved in both groups	Improved in both groups	Improved in both groups	Improved in both groups
QOL	Improved	Improved	Improved in both groups	Improved in both groups	Improved in both groups	Improved in both groups	Improved in both groups
Major Adverse events	Infection, bleeding device failure 2.35 times higher in HM XVE	Bleeding, stroke, infection, device failure higher in HM 2	Disabling stroke, re-operation for device failure less in HM 2	Bleeding, infection, stroke, device failure similar	More stroke, less device failure in HVAD	Re-operation for device failure less in HM 3	Re-operation for device failure, stroke less in HM 3

Abbreviations: INTERMACS, Interagency Registry for Mechanically Assisted Circulatory Support; OMT, optimal medical therapy; QOL, quality of life; TX, transplantation.

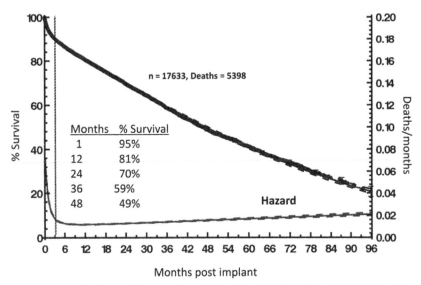

Intermᵃcs **Continuous Flow LVAD/BiVAD Implants: 2008 – 2016, n = 17633**

Fig. 2. Parametric survival curve from INTERMACS Registry for CF-LVADs, including both iso-lated LVADs and BiVAD stratified by INTERMACS profile at the time of implant. The dashed lines indicate 70% confidence limits. (*From* Kirklin JK, Pagani FD, Kormos RL, et al. Eighth annual INTERMACS report: special focus on framing the impact of adverse events. J Heart Lung Transplant 2017;36(10):1081; with permission.)

Although usually LVADs are implanted as either BTT or DT, a significant proportion of patients also receives an LVAD, as a BTD.[8] As an example, LVADs have been effec-tive in lowering pulmonary pressures and pulmonary vascular resistance to permis-sible levels in patients with advanced HF and World Health Organization group 2

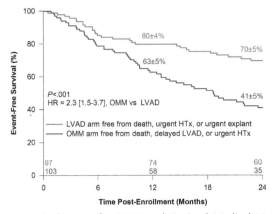

Fig. 3. Kaplan-Meier survival curves for LVAD and Optimal Medical Management (OMM) arm from the ROADMAP Study. HR, hazard ratio. (*From* Starling RC, Estep JD, Horstmanshof DA, et al. Risk assessment and comparative effectiveness of left ventricular assist device and medical management in ambulatory heart failure patients: the ROADMAP study 2-year re-sults. JACC Heart Fail 2017;5(7):521; with permission.)

pulmonary hypertension with unacceptably high PVR despite optimal medical therapy, allowing them to become more suitable HT candidates.[9] Another example includes LVADs for marginal transplant candidates who would otherwise be waiting for a long time on the UNOS transplant waiting list because of large body mass or unfavorable blood group type. A third example is patients who present in INTERMACS profile 1 and need emergent LVAD implantation, before their candidacy for transplantation can be assessed.

The 1-year survival on LVAD therapy is starting to rival that observed after HT. The 3-year survival and beyond however falls short of what is seen with HT, although most patients who survive 3 years on LVAD therapy receive the device for a DT indication. Advances in engineering and improved understanding of flow mechanics have already shown a significant decline in complications such as pump thrombosis and need for reoperation for device replacement with the newest generation of HeartMate III (Thoratec, Pleasanton, CA, USA) LVAD. Whether LVAD therapy will be offered as an alternative to HT in the future remains to be seen. Risk stratification to choose between HT and LVAD therapies for specific patients to allow for maximal quality and length of life will become the key challenge in the coming years.

FOCUS ON PATIENT-CENTERED CARE AND QUALITY OF LIFE

In patients suffering from end-stage HF, LVADs offer a chance at improved quality of life, albeit not as much when compared with HT. However, if LVAD therapy is to become an increasingly used option in patients with ambulatory HF, its impact on quality of life will become a major driver in decision making. In each patient, the potential to improve the survival and quality of life for patients and their families must be weighed against numerous potential complications and burdens related to this therapy. Providing patient-centered care requires that the short- and long-term risks and benefits of therapy are understood, appropriate patient selection is focused on, timing of implantation is optimized, as well as the risk-benefit profiles of this therapy are individualized in each patient.[10]

Rehospitalization following LVAD implantation has a major impact on the overall quality of life, for the patient as well as for their caregivers.[8] In a recent systematic review, adverse events in the year following DT LVAD implementation were 55% for rehospitalization, 30% for major bleeding, 20% for device-related infection, and 10% for disabling stroke.[11] Any measures that help reduce pump-associated adverse events, and hence, rehospitalizations, would lower that burden immensely. Currently approved continuous flow devices are superior to the previous pulsatile LVADs in terms of survival and risk of adverse events.[12,13] The newer-generation devices allow for pulsatility and rotary designs that allow for even smaller profiles and improved durability. Less important, yet a meaningful impact on quality of life is perceived by the weight and bulk of associated batteries and controller, which it is hoped will continue to improve in size and duration of battery life in the coming years. A transcutaneous or alternative source of energy that allows patients to disengage from their drivelines for increasing amounts of time would be a major step in improving lifestyle. Future engineering improvements must focus not only on improved long-term event-free survival but also on improved quality of life for both patients and caregivers, by facilitating self-care and independence and reducing reliance on caregivers.

FOCUS ON MYOCARDIAL RECOVERY AND ROLE OF CONCOMITANT MEDICAL THERAPY

Using LVAD as a BTR is a promising option, especially in select patients with nonischemic cardiomyopathy. Typically noted in patients with acute onset of myocardial dysfunction, such as peripartum cardiomyopathy or myocarditis, it is made feasible by evidence-based adjunctive pharmacologic therapies. Recovery in patients with ischemic cardiomyopathy is much rarer, given the extent of infarction usually involved to cause end-stage HF necessitating an LVAD implantation. Initially reported as anecdotal cases, myocardial recovery gained focus after Birks and colleagues[14] reported a successful explant strategy in preselected young patients with nonischemic cardiomyopathy. In their study, 73.3% of the patients (total 15) implanted with durable LVAD (HeartMate XVE, Thoratec, Pleasanton, CA, USA) and treated with neurohormonal blockade and clenbuterol exhibited myocardial recovery, including normalization of left ventricular ejection fraction (LVEF) and the ability to explant the device. In a subsequent study, they demonstrated a similarly high recovery rate (63%) in preselected patients with continuous flow devices as well.[15,16] Dandel and colleagues[16] reported a post-explant survival of 65% to 75% at 10 years, with a 35% to 45% chance of recurrence of HF. Since then, multiple single-center experiences on myocardial recovery have reported wide ranges of rates of recovery.

However, an analysis of INTERMACS data confirms that the overall rate of myocardial recovery on LVAD support is rather low at 1.3%.[17] There is a subgroup of patients with a higher rate of myocardial recovery, characterized by age less than 50 years, nonischemic cause, HF less than 2 years, lack of implantable cardioverter-defibrillator, creatinine less than 1.2 mg/dL, and LV end-diastolic diameter less than 6.5 cm.[18] The wide variability in the observations may be related to the fact that there is inconsistency in the definition of myocardial recovery. A framework for myocardial recovery on LVAD support has been proposed (**Fig. 4**).[19] It is hoped the results from the RESTAGE-HF (Remission from Stage D Heart Failure; Clinical Trial NCT01774656) will help clarify this further. It is imperative to try and differentiate between reverse

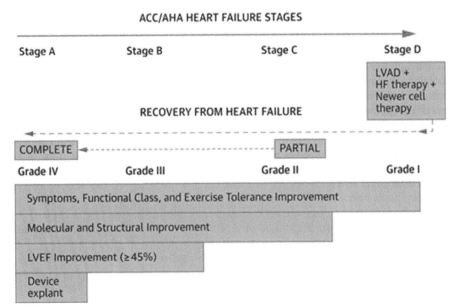

Fig. 4. Proposed framework for myocardial recovery on LVAD support juxtaposed with American College of Cardiology/American Heart Association stages of HF. HTx, heart transplantation. (*From* Agarwal R, Murali S. Recovering the broken-hearted: the ultimate (and uncertain) goal of mechanical circulatory support. J Am Coll Cardiol 2016;68(16):1754; with permission.)

remodeling, which may represent a "remission" of the myocardial failure and actual myocardial recovery before proceeding with an LVAD explant, given that improvement in LVEF does not always imply that the underlying cellular biology and pathophysiology has also returned to normal. In the coming years, stem cell therapy, including endogenous cardiac or pluripotent stem cells in addition to medical therapy, may allow for cell repair and regeneration.

In the vast majority of patients, however, LVADs are implanted as BTT or DT, without hope for meaningful myocardial recovery. In these patients, little is known about the role of concomitant medical therapy, except for its role in management of comorbidities such as systemic hypertension. It is unknown if LVAD patients would necessarily benefit from neurohormonal blockade, which is the mainstay of evidence-based therapy in HFrEF.

FOCUS ON RISK STRATIFICATION

Patient selection is a key determinant of clinical outcomes with LVAD therapy. A better understanding of the patient profile that derives the most benefit from LVAD technology has allowed improved survival outcomes. This change is exemplified by a noticeable drop in the INTERMACS profile 1 patient from 44% to 14% in recent years, with a simultaneous improvement in survival each year.[20] Because HF is a heterogeneous condition, risk stratification needs to be both sophisticated and individualized for consistent optimal outcomes with LVAD therapy.

A host of risk scores for LVAD implantation has been developed and validated to aid the clinician in appropriate patient selection.[21–26] Although there are published guidelines for patient selection for HT, there is limited guidance for patient selection for LVAD therapy. Current guidelines from the International Society of Heart and Lung Transplantation recommend that HF patients who are at "high risk for 1-year mortality using prognostic models" should be referred for advanced therapies as appropriate (class II a, level of evidence C). Although the guidelines do not specify any particular prognostic models, the current selection is limited. Validated tools, such as the Seattle Heart Failure model and the Heart Failure Survival Score, tend to underestimate absolute risk and overestimate survival in end-stage HF. New York Heart Association classification, although commonly used in HF, is subjective, inconsistent, and susceptible to significant interobserver variability. The INTERMACS profile of the patient at the time of LVAD implantation allows for prognostic discrimination, with INTERMACS profile 1 patients having the worst outcomes.[23] The HeartMate II risk score (HMRS) was introduced as a measure to predict 90-day and 1-year mortality in patients receiving a continuous flow HeartMate II (Thoratec, Pleasanton, CA, USA) LVAD.[24] It was derived from and validated within 1122 patients enrolled in the original HeartMate II clinical trials. Although simplistic and easy to calculate, its applicability in routine clinical practice has been quite limited in the diverse population of patients being considered for contemporary LVADs.[25] Machine learning methods using Bayesian analysis can overcome some of the limitations of existing risk scores and are being evaluated for risk stratification for both mortality and major adverse events after LVAD implantation.[27] This risk stratification model is an improvement over HMRS and maintains its accuracy irrespective of device type or device indication. Future integration of this risk tool with electronic health records will allow for easy, rapid risk assessment at the bedside, which will greatly enhance patient selection and clinical decision making for LVAD therapy.

FOCUS ON PULSATILITY AND FLOW

In patients being implanted with CF-LVADs, continuous flow physiology reduces arterial pulse pressure and pulsatility to an extent that is unique to this population.

Reduced pulsatility may contribute to ischemic and hemorrhagic stroke, vascular dysfunction, increased oxidative stress, development of arteriovenous malformations, especially in the gastrointestinal tract, as well as increased aortic stiffness. The clinical outcomes with CF-LVADs are clearly superior to Pulsatile-LVADs, and the latter are no longer used in clinical practice. The newest generation of CF-LVADs (HeartMate III and HVAD) offers centrifugal flow instead of axial flow, and these devices are less prone to pump thrombosis and the need for device replacement.[28] Device interrogation with optimization of flow and pulsatility is needed to maximize benefit of LVAD therapy in each patient. It is hoped that future generations of LVAD will allow for automation of pulsatility and flow tailored to the patient's needs at any given time.

FOCUS ON COST-EFFECTIVENESS OF DURABLE LEFT VENTRICULAR ASSIST DEVICES

The cost for HF care continues to increase placing a heavy burden on the US health care system. The overall cost of HF care was $30.9 billion in 2012 and is expected to increase to $43.6 billion in 2020 and $63.7 billion in 2030. Frequent hospitalization, particularly in those patients with advanced disease, is a key driver of the total cost. The incremental cost-effectiveness ratio (ICER) is a statistic used in cost-effectiveness analysis in health care to summarize the cost-effectiveness of an intervention. It is defined by the difference in cost between 2 interventions, divided by the difference in their effect. The quality-adjusted life-year (QALY) is a summary measure of health outcome for economic evaluation, which incorporates the impact on both the quantity and the quality of life. In a recent analysis of 220 Medicare beneficiaries with HF, the mean cost of LVAD implantation was $175,420. The cost of readmission was lower before LVAD implant when compared with after LVAD therapy, although outpatient monthly costs were similar. LVAD increased QALYs, readmissions, and costs compared with medical management, yielding an ICER of $209,400 per QALY gained.[29] It therefore appears that cost-effectiveness of LVAD therapy is not favorable except in low-risk subgroups who have fewer readmissions and less frequent hospitalizations. Identification of the right patient and LVAD implantation at the right time before the HF becomes very severe is needed to improve cost-effectiveness of LVAD therapy.

FOCUS ON MINIMALLY INVASIVE IMPLANTATION TECHNIQUES

The past several years have shown an increased interest in less invasive approaches to LVAD implantation. Potential advantages include less bleeding and coagulopathy, easier postoperative recovery, avoidance of right ventricular (RV) dysfunction, reduced length of hospital stay, and safer sternal reentry at time of transplantation.[30] These theories have been investigated in small series, multi-institutional database reviews, and a single prospective observational trial.[31–34]

A variety of techniques have been described for HeartMate II, HeartWare (HeartWare, Framingham, MA, USA) HVAD, and HeartMate III implantation. The most common surgical strategy involves partial sternotomy with left thoracotomy using either central or peripheral cannulation for cardiopulmonary bypass. LVAD inflow is obtained via the left ventricular (LV) apex, and outflow is to the ascending aorta. Sternal-sparing techniques have also been described with the outflow graft being sewn to either the ascending aorta (via right mini thoracotomy) or the axillary artery. Off-pump implantation is feasible and relies on completion of all surgical steps, including driveline tunneling, outflow graft anastomosis, and deairing before apical coring. Apical coring is accomplished during rapid ventricular pacing to minimize blood loss and facilitate efficient insertion of the LVAD inflow. Thoratec's HeartMate III has been designed to be placed entirely intrathoracic, whereas the HVAD LATERAL Study is designed to test nonsternotomy techniques of full-support ventricular assist device (VAD) implantation.[35] The next generation of pump, HeartWare's MVAD, is an even smaller pump that can be placed via a minimally invasive procedure.[34]

It is worth noting that even these "less invasive" techniques are not entirely "minimally invasive." A significant thoracotomy with muscle splitting and rib spreading is required because of the profile of even the smallest pumps currently available. Small thoracic incisions may make direct access to the LV apex technically more challenging and result in improper placement of the inflow cannula. Similarly, limited exposure/access to the ascending aorta may encumber emergent cardiopulmonary bypass if needed.[30] The feasibility and safety of minimally invasive LVAD implantation in appropriate patients are fairly established, and outcomes will continue to improve with refinement of technology with newer-generation pumps.

FOCUS ON DURABLE BIVENTRICULAR SUPPORT

The incidence of RV dysfunction requiring right ventricular assist device (RVAD) after LVAD implantation has been reported between 5% and 20%.[1] These patients face a higher mortality than those with durable LVAD support only. Preoperative optimization of the RV with medical therapy has led to better patient outcomes. However, RV dysfunction that is unable to be managed with medical therapy continues to be a vexing issue. Although early, planned use of mechanical support for the RV is associated with improved survival, the most effective and safest BiVAD device configuration remains unknown. Options for short- to medium-term support include Abbott Centrimag, Abiomed Impella, and TandemHeart Protek Duo.

The Centrimag device consists of an extracorporeal, magnetically levitated blood pump that can provide RV, LV, or extracorporeal membrane oxygenation (ECMO) support, depending on cannulation strategy and the presence or absence of an oxygenator in the circuit. RVAD support with a Centrimag is usually configured with transcutaneous cannulas: right atrial venous drainage and pulmonary arterial outflow via sternotomy. Strategies have been developed, with femoral venous drainage and a cannulated graft to the pulmonary artery (PA) that can facilitate discontinuation of RV support without the need for resternotomy. The device can be combined with an oxygenator to provide respiratory ECMO support in conjunction with support of the RV. This setup can be maintained for weeks with low rates of hemolysis and excellent support. Patients can be ambulated but must be maintained in the hospital.

The Abiomed Impella is a percutaneous axial flow device inserted via the femoral vein. The pump is housed in a long flexible catheter and sits in the RV outflow tract with the catheter traversing the pulmonic valve and delivering flow to the PA. The device has been approved for short-term RV support and has benefits including ease of implant via a truly percutaneous approach. Limitations include the inability to ambulate or to use an oxygenator with the system as well as positional instability and hemolysis. The Tandem Life Protek Duo is a specialized cannula designed to facilitate RV support. It can be placed either via the femoral or internal jugular vein and traverses the right heart terminating in the PA under fluoroscopic guidance. It is driven by the Tandem Life extracorporeal pump. A bearing in the pump requires heparinized saline infusion to prevent heat generation.

Longer-term options for durable biventricular support include Syncardia Total Artificial Heart or placement of durable VAD, such as HeartWare HVAD for both left and right ventricles.[36] Outcomes in these very ill patients are generally inferior to patients who receive isolated LVAD support reflecting the severity of biventricular failure, limitations of current technology, and surgical challenges. Challenges with dual VAD support also include lack of domain for the device or devices in the chest and difficulties balancing right- and left-sided flow with separate controllers.

FOCUS ON FULLY IMPLANTABLE SYSTEMS

One of the main limitations of current VAD technology is the percutaneous driveline, which can be a source of discomfort to the patients as well as a nidus for infection. Driveline infections range from local and superficial, to deep-seated device infection with systemic sepsis and risk of death. A great deal of effort has been dedicated to technology allowing transcutaneous energy transfer (TET). TET can transmit electrical power to an implanted device without skin penetration relying on inductive coupling with transmitter and receiver coils. The potential to realize fully implantable "wireless" LVAD with TET technology will improve as LVADs become smaller and do not require a volume displacement chamber, and the engineering behind TET improves. With further LVAD miniaturization and lower power requirements, a totally implantable system using a reliable energy transfer system should be realized in the foreseeable future. The first applications may be seen in smaller, partial support devices (needing less power) for less ill patients requiring less than full cardiac support.

SUMMARY

LVADs have revolutionized the treatment options for patients suffering from advanced HF. As the patient population that can benefit from this technology expands, it is imperative for caregivers and medical professionals to keep abreast of the practices to minimize complications and anticipate roadblocks to overcome. As patient survival continues to improve, the reduction of morbidity and improvement of quality of life have taken precedence in leading the drive for further and future improvements.

REFERENCES

1. Kirklin JK, Pagani FD, Kormos RL, et al. Eighth annual INTERMACS report: special focus on framing the impact of adverse events. J Heart Lung Transplant 2017;36(10):1080–6.
2. Stewart GC, Givertz MM. Mechanical circulatory support for advanced heart failure: patients and technology in evolution. Circulation 2012;125(10):1304–15.
3. Ammirati E, Oliva FG, Colombo T, et al. Mid-term survival after continuous-flow left ventricular assist device versus heart transplantation. Heart Vessels 2016;31(5): 722–33.
4. Schumer EM, Black MC, Monreal G, et al. Left ventricular assist devices: current controversies and future directions. Eur Heart J 2016;37(46):3434–9.
5. Lee DS, Gona P, Vasan RS, et al. Relation of disease etiology and risk factors to heart failure with preserved ejection fraction or reduced ejection fraction: insights from the National Heart, Lung, and Blood Institute's Framingham Heart Study. Circulation 2009;119(24):3070–7.
6. Grupper A, Park SJ, Pereira NL, et al. Role of ventricular assist therapy for patients with heart failure and restrictive physiology: improving outcomes for a lethal disease. J Heart Lung Transplant 2015;34(8):1042–9.
7. Starling RC, Estep JD, Horstmanshof DA, et al. Risk assessment and comparative effectiveness of left ventricular assist device and medical management in ambulatory heart failure patients: the ROADMAP study 2-year results. JACC Heart Fail 2017;5(7):518–27.

8. Stehlik J, Stevenson LW, Edwards LB, et al. Organ allocation around the world: insights from the ISHLT International Registry for Heart and Lung Transplantation. J Heart Lung Transplant 2014;33(10):975–84.
9. Raina A, Kanwar M. New drugs and devices in the pipeline for heart failure with reduced ejection fraction versus heart failure with preserved ejection fraction. Curr Heart Fail Rep 2014;11(4):374–81.
10. Breathett K, Allen LA, Ambardekar AV. Patient-centered care for left ventricular assist device therapy: current challenges and future directions. Curr Opin Cardiol 2016;31(3):313–20.
11. McIlvennan CK, Magid KH, Ambardekar AV, et al. Clinical outcomes after continuous-flow left ventricular assist device: a systematic review. Circ Heart Fail 2014;7(6):1003–13.
12. Slaughter MS, Rogers JG, Milano CA, et al. Advanced heart failure treated with continuous-flow left ventricular assist device. N Engl J Med 2009;361(23):2241–51.
13. Aaronson KD, Slaughter MS, Miller LW, et al. Use of an intrapericardial, continuous-flow, centrifugal pump in patients awaiting heart transplantation. Circulation 2012;125(25):3191–200.
14. Birks EJ, Tansley PD, Hardy J, et al. Left ventricular assist device and drug therapy for the reversal of heart failure. N Engl J Med 2006;355(18):1873–84.
15. Birks EJ, George RS, Hedger M, et al. Reversal of severe heart failure with a continuous-flow left ventricular assist device and pharmacological therapy: a prospective study. Circulation 2011;123(4):381–90.
16. Dandel M, Weng Y, Siniawski H, et al. Prediction of cardiac stability after weaning from left ventricular assist devices in patients with idiopathic dilated cardiomyopathy. Circulation 2008;118(14 Suppl):S94–105.
17. Kirklin JK, Naftel DC, Pagani FD, et al. Sixth INTERMACS annual report: a 10,000-patient database. J Heart Lung Transplant 2014;33(6):555–64.
18. Wever-Pinzon O, Drakos SG, McKellar SH, et al. Cardiac recovery during long-term left ventricular assist device support. J Am Coll Cardiol 2016;68(14):1540–53.
19. Agarwal R, Murali S. Recovering the broken-hearted: the ultimate (and uncertain) goal of mechanical circulatory support. J Am Coll Cardiol 2016;68(16):1753–5.
20. Kirklin JK, Naftel DC, Pagani FD, et al. Seventh INTERMACS annual report: 15,000 patients and counting. J Heart Lung Transplant 2015;34(12):1495–504.
21. Cowger JA, Castle L, Aaronson KD, et al. The HeartMate II risk score: an adjusted score for evaluation of all continuous-flow left ventricular assist devices. ASAIO J 2016;62(3):281–5.
22. Drakos SG, Janicki L, Horne BD, et al. Risk factors predictive of right ventricular failure after left ventricular assist device implantation. Am J Cardiol 2010;105(7):1030–5.
23. Loghmanpour NA, Kormos RL, Kanwar MK, et al. A Bayesian model to predict right ventricular failure following left ventricular assist device therapy. JACC Heart Fail 2016;4(9):711–21.
24. Cowger J, Sundareswaran K, Rogers JG, et al. Predicting survival in patients receiving continuous flow left ventricular assist devices: the HeartMate II risk score. J Am Coll Cardiol 2013;61(3):313–21.
25. Kanwar MK, Lohmueller LC, Kormos RL, et al. Low accuracy of the HeartMate risk score for predicting mortality using the INTERMACS registry data. ASAIO J 2017;63(3):251–6.

26. Boyle AJ, Ascheim DD, Russo MJ, et al. Clinical outcomes for continuous-flow left ventricular assist device patients stratified by pre-operative INTERMACS classification. J Heart Lung Transplant 2011;30(4):402–7.
27. Loghmanpour NA, Kanwar MK, Druzdzel MJ, et al. A new Bayesian network-based risk stratification model for prediction of short-term and long-term LVAD mortality. ASAIO J 2015;61(3):313–23.
28. Mehra MR, Naka Y, Uriel N, et al. A fully magnetically levitated circulatory pump for advanced heart failure. N Engl J Med 2017;376(5):440–50.
29. Baras SJ, Goldhaber-Fiebert JD, Banerjee D, et al. Cost-effectiveness of left ventricular assist devices in ambulatory patients with advanced heart failure. JACC Heart Fail 2017;5(2):110–9.
30. Patil NP, Popov AF, Simon AR. Minimally invasive left ventricular assist device implantation: at the crossroads. J Thorac Dis 2015;7(4):564–5.
31. Strueber M, Meyer AL, Feussner M, et al. A minimally invasive off-pump implantation technique for continuous-flow left ventricular assist devices: early experience. J Heart Lung Transplant 2014;33(8):851–6.
32. Haberl T, Riebandt J, Mahr S, et al. Viennese approach to minimize the invasiveness of ventricular assist device implantation†. Eur J Cardiothorac Surg 2014; 46(6):991–6 [discussion: 996].
33. Popov AF, Hosseini MT, Zych B, et al. HeartWare left ventricular assist device implantation through bilateral anterior thoracotomy. Ann Thorac Surg 2012;93(2): 674–6.
34. Rojas SV, Avsar M, Hanke JS, et al. Minimally invasive ventricular assist device surgery. Artif Organs 2015;39(6):473–9.
35. Kilic A. The future of left ventricular assist devices. J Thorac Dis 2015;7(12): 2188–93.
36. Kirklin JK. Advances in mechanical assist devices and artificial hearts for children. Curr Opin Pediatr 2015;27(5):597–603.

Moving?

Make sure your subscription moves with you!

To notify us of your new address, find your **Clinics Account Number** (located on your mailing label above your name), and contact customer service at:

Email: journalscustomerservice-usa@elsevier.com

800-654-2452 (subscribers in the U.S. & Canada)
314-447-8871 (subscribers outside of the U.S. & Canada)

Fax number: 314-447-8029

**Elsevier Health Sciences Division
Subscription Customer Service
3251 Riverport Lane
Maryland Heights, MO 63043**

*To ensure uninterrupted delivery of your subscription, please notify us at least 4 weeks in advance of move.